Breaking the Power of Addiction

Daily Readings in Recovery from Addiction

by Dr Chris Noble

Published by New Generation Publishing in 2022

Copyright © Dr Chris Noble 2022

First Edition

The author asserts the moral right under the Copyright, Designs and Patents Act 1988 to be identified as the author of this work.

All Rights reserved. No part of this publication may be reproduced, stored in a retrieval system or transmitted, in any form or by any means without the prior consent of the author, nor be otherwise circulated in any form of binding or cover other than that which it is published and without a similar condition being imposed on the subsequent purchaser.

ISBN   978-1-80369-237-1

www.newgeneration-publishing.com

New Generation Publishing

Introduction

These daily readings come from my own journey out from the grip of addiction and into a life of freedom from the compulsion to drink alcohol.

Using my own story of a life-long battle to break free from my addiction to alcohol and then my journey into recovery, I have sought to expose both the complexity and the spiritual nature of this most perplexing condition.

For years I tried to understand my drinking because I thought that if I could understand it then I would be able to bring it under control. I tried many ways out including religion and even became a priest, but that didn't work either. Controlled drinking brought less control and it wasn't until I met other drinkers like me who were seeking to break free from its grip, that I finally found a way out.

These readings chronicle my own journey out of the darkness of the power of addiction and into the light of recovery.

I hope you will find them helpful for your journey especially if you or a loved one is caught in the snare of addiction to alcohol or anything else.

January

1.1 Doing the Job

There are a lot of us, people who like a drink. We wouldn't want to put a label on ourselves, but in our more reflective moments, we know that our drinking is an issue. We have job's, careers, families, churches and much besides. We might not even drink every day, so what's the problem? Why not just carry on?

My epiphany came one day in the pub. I was drinking at the bar with a friend who was necking neat vodkas. I said 'do you always drink like that?' She said 'yes.' I said 'why?' And she said, 'because it does the job.'

It was as if someone had held a mirror up to my drinking. All the façade and smokescreen of respectability that I had surrounded my drinking with, fell away. I saw that in a slightly more sophisticated way I was doing the same thing. My drinking was doing the job, but what job was it doing?

My friend at the bar died a few years later as a consequence of this disease and I often think of her as I go out to help others who are in trouble with their drinking. Without her even knowing it she introduced me to a life of recovery and as a result I have received my freedom and a life that I never thought possible.

1.2 City Drinking

When I worked in the City of London, someone used the term alcohol abuse in a conversation at the wine bar in the basement of our office building. Dressed in our smart suites and business clothes we seemed a million miles away from the street drinkers who hung around the doorways of the city churches. The words alcohol abuse raised a jeer and a call for another round of drinks.

With the benefit of hindsight, I can see that without knowing it many of us had unwittingly crossed some invisible line into problem drinking. Not everyone in our group would go on to develop a full-blown drink problem and for some like myself, it would take many years to realise that I had a habit that was impacting my life in a very negative way.

The champagne and oyster bars with their impressive décor and subtle lighting made drinking seem so normal and respectable. What could possibly be wrong with a few cool beers and some champagne on ice?

The answer is that there could be quite a lot wrong with a few beers let alone the champagne. I used to have a few beers every night after work in the city. I'd also had a few beers at lunchtime so it seemed quite natural to continue after work. Of course, those few beers were rarely few and they usually became many.

Innocent fun? Maybe, but these few beers set in place patterns of drinking that came back to haunt me.

My weekends would revolve around drinking in pubs and going to parties where there was more drinking. Without realising it I laid down a pattern of extreme drinking that was hardwired into me in a way that I did not appreciate at the time.

It was all so normal and there was nothing alarming or concerning about it. After all, what's wrong with a few beers?

1.3 In the Family

The drinking culture of the City of London was foreshadowed for me as I grew up in a home where drinking was a problem. I don't see myself as a victim but I now realise that my father's binge drinking had a significant effect on our home life and my upbringing.

I don't understand my father's drinking or the effect that it had on him, but for me, I felt uneasy and fearful in our house as anger could flare up at any moment. What my father's rage deposited in me was a constant feeling of insecurity and fear as I lived under the shadow of the next 'good clout.' Ironically it was this fear and insecurity that set the stage for my own dependence on alcohol.

Our family story of appalling poverty and unemployment in a deeply working-class area of Tyneside in the North East of England provided the ideal environment for hard drinking to thrive. Alcoholism has a long history in my family that goes back many generations most notably to a very dubious and notorious character called 'blackbird'.

In spite of starting so far back my father was a fine man who achieved a huge amount in his life. I loved him dearly, but he died without ever figuring out what was wrong. I can't say for sure but I think he had a form of this disease and the 'ism' that comes with it. He rarely showed his hand, but I still remember one phone call shortly after he retired when he was truly honest with me and said, 'I'm desperate.' Following that he never mentioned it again, but it gave me a tiny glimpse through the tightly shut window of his heart.

I can now see that he battled with it, and for large parts of his life he overcame it.

1.4 Early Warning Signs

As an eleven-year-old, I attended a youth group that met on Tuesday evenings in the sports hall of a local school. The people who ran it arranged team games and we used to run around until we were all exhausted. At halftime, they would open a 'tuck shop' which sold sweets and cola drinks. The sweets were cheap, very sugary and I would buy and eat lots of them. Every week I would eat the sweets and drink the coke until I felt sick.

I could not control my input and every week I would say to myself that I will never do that again. I would vow to go easy on the sweets and the coke but I could not control my consumption, and the next week I would once again get my fill and feel very sick as a result.

I've thought about this quite a lot and I have wondered if this was just an early warning sign of what was to happen with my drinking. Looking back, I can see that it was the same pattern of excess, loss of control and sickness that came later in life through my drinking. Perhaps it was an early warning sign.

The youth group was a religious one and even though my parents were non-religious they sent me every Sunday. Because I went for fifty Sundays in a year, I was awarded a special bible and Sir Cliff Richard made the presentation.

I still have that bible and although I didn't really understand what it was all about, I was blessed by the friendliness and encouragement of those folks. What I saw in them was a different way of living, a spiritual one.

There was of course not a whiff of booze amongst them, although Sir Cliff went on to buy a vineyard in Portugal.

1.5 The Elixir of Life

At thirteen years of age, I had two shots of vodka. The effect was instantaneous and wonderful. All my fear evaporated. I felt that I had found the elixir of life. My social anxieties lifted and I felt that I was at one with the universe. It was a sort of spiritual experience and a moment of enlightenment.

I'm pretty sure that not everyone who takes their first strong drink experiences this kind of thing so what was going on? Why did I have such a huge reaction to this substance? It really was mind-blowing, so much so that I can remember it vividly all these years later. I think the answer is that I was predisposed to alcohol in a way that normal people are not. Alcohol did something in me that it doesn't do in a lot of other people.

I did not know at the time or for many years to come that my exceptionally euphoric response to alcohol was an indicator that I was a potential alcoholic.

From that day onwards I was chasing the high that I had experienced from the vodka shots. That day alcohol gave me such a temporary sense of wellbeing and peace that all I wanted was to feel like that again.

I now see that on that day my potential alcoholism had been activated and the clock had started ticking. From that day onwards I began to crave my next drink. It wasn't long before I found it and many more besides.

1.6 Social Lubricant

I liked the way that alcohol took away my fear, particularly my fear of people. I found that with a drink inside I could fit in and feel like I belonged to any group of people.

All I had to do to be part of my social group was to drink, it was that simple, that easy. Alcohol helped me and drinking made me feel that I belonged. It gave me a sense that I was part of, rather than outside, any particular social gathering.

I found that with alcohol, I could lose my inhibitions and even be the life and soul of the party. Alcohol enabled me to break out of my natural shyness and reserve releasing my alter-ego. Alcohol worked for me as a shy teenager as it enabled me to socialise, be confident and overcome my adolescent social anxiety.

Alcohol is a wonderful social lubricant and I guess that is why we use it in our culture as an ice breaker to help people to loosen up a bit and get the party going. However, when it came to social events, I was much more dependent on alcohol than my friends were. I needed it to get me up and running whereas many of my friends could function perfectly well in social situations without it.

1.7 Escape Artist

I still have my earliest school report from when I was five years old which said that I daydreamed and didn't get on with my work. I was a dreamer and as I got older, I lived more and more inside my own head.

This escape from reality just kept on developing especially with drinking. I found that alcohol enabled me to escape from my worries and deeply seated fears. Reality can be tough and escape via the bottle was an attractive and easy option for me. I drank in order to escape myself, my feelings and the realities of life that I didn't like. My drinking was escapism, pure and simple.

When I took a drink, I could put my life on hold and disengage from reality so that I didn't have to feel the external pressure of living in the real world.

I totally identify with the addicts and alcoholics at our local detox centre. I share their desire to escape from reality, but their devastated health is a constant reminder to me that alcoholic escapism is not a long-term solution to life's problems, however difficult and distressing they may be.

I know from experience that the reality we seek to escape from becomes the very thing that binds us and ties us up. Alcohol offers freedom but in actual fact just produces bondage and imprisonment in the cycle of addiction.

1.8 Survival Tactics

Growing up in a drinking household meant that I had to learn to protect myself both physically and emotionally, so I developed a number of survival tactics. The insecurity of my home deposited within me a constant feeling that something was just about to go wrong.

It was difficult to enjoy good times because I was always haunted by the thought that things were too good and something bad was about to happen. I always had to be on guard and ready for the next crisis which meant that I found it difficult to relax and I was stressed out a lot.

One very important survival technique was never to express an opinion or let on about how I was really feeling. The sharing of feelings within my home was confined to outbursts of anger from my father and tears of fear from my mother. So, my heart learned never to share my feelings or thinking with those close to me and I either buried my emotions, hid my thoughts or shared with people who were outside the family.

This survival tactic worked in my dysfunctional home but the protection mechanism remained deeply entrenched in my life and has caused me problems as I have struggled to share my feelings and thinking with those closest to me.

1.9 New Society

One person who I was able to talk with was my friend's dad who was an antique dealer and also a radical political thinker. We used to sit in the kitchen of his house in Tunbridge Wells drinking coffee, smoking and talking about revolutionary social change.

He introduced me to 'New Society' magazine and those conversations around the kitchen table were formative in my life as they gave me an altruistic vision that had not been part of my life at home.

He wasn't a drinker but he knew all about it from his military service in the Coldstream Guards. I think his class war philosophy rubbed off on me more than I realised as he planted some important ideas in me that have had a governing underlying effect in my life.

He managed to communicate to me the importance of not living for yourself only and those conversations were influential in my decisions to live a life not based purely on materialistic considerations.

I remember that he also took me to church on Christmas Eve when I was worse for wear. I came round in the middle of the midnight service, feeling sick, wondering where I was and how I got there. I always think of that now when I take the midnight service at Christmas. I have been there.

1.10 Subversive Drinking

Obtaining and drinking alcohol in my teenage years was for me a subversive activity. In the early days, it was against the rules and when I managed to get hold of alcohol there was a sense of victory over the system. Getting drunk had a rebellious and subversive feel and I enjoyed being part of the drinking culture.

At school, drinking gave me an identity as one of the cool people who drank and smoked, and I liked that. We compared ourselves to the straight people who didn't drink or smoke. We were anti-establishment and didn't want to play the game of life as it seemed to be set out. So instead, we drank and gravitated towards the music scene as we pursued what we thought was an alternative lifestyle.

It was a nice idea but it was just an illusion and instead of finding freedom I was just getting further into slavery to alcohol and other things that were to have a negative impact on the whole course of my life. We all thought that we were so cool with our long hair and flared trousers and in a way, we were, but only for a season.

The long-term fallout has been pretty brutal with early deaths, cancers, overdoses, mental hospitals, homelessness and prison.

I have been spared some of these more extreme consequences and I am thankful for that. I no longer need to be cool and I can put my subversive disposition to good use in trying to change things that need to be changed.

1.11 Boot Camp

Public school life in the early 1970s was tough. It was dirty, noisy, violent and unsafe, especially for an immature child. It was a relief to be away from the conflict in my family home but it was a case of out of the frying pan and into the fire. There were a lot of other boys from troubled or broken homes who like me were confused and emotionally messed up.

I was always in a state of heightened anxiety at school and since I was a boarder that meant that it was difficult to relax or detach from the situation. It was a bit like being in the military where you have to keep your kit on and your weapon with you at all times in case of attack.

It seems hard to believe that punishment for minor infringements of the school rules was administered through beatings with a cane.

I don't think school was too dissimilar from being in prison. It was very Darwinian as it was based on the survival of the fittest. Somehow, I managed to carve out a niche in the structure and I survived, although by the time I left I had been well educated in vice.

1.12 Risky Rocky Places

As a teenager, I used to gravitate toward a pub called the Sussex Arms near the Pantiles in Tunbridge Wells. This was pre-punk, in the latter stages of the hippie era, and it was a popular venue for young people seeking an alternative lifestyle in the drug and music culture of the time.

One evening we all left the pub and went back to a squat where somebody went crazy and stabbed me in the arm with a knife. There was no reason for this apart from the effect that the alcohol and drugs were having. I was taken to hospital and the knife wound in my arm was stitched up. I thought little of it at the time but it was really just another early warning sign about the risky and dangerous places that alcohol was to take me. Even today I still get mild pain on the site of that knife wound.

This didn't put me off risky, rocky places and after leaving school I played the drums in a local rock band performing in pubs and clubs. Having a few drinks inside helped me to relax and I found it easier to get into the groove. Music and drinking became inseparably linked and certain types of music seemed to stir up my desire to drink.

Years later when I was playing drums in a local rock band, I sometimes felt that the music was inciting people to debauchery which would have been okay except for the fact that I was the Vicar!

1.13 Mythologies

Alcoholism is not just about how much you drink. It's much deeper than that. It's a disease with many different stages that can manifest in different ways. Many alcoholics like myself do not conform to the stereotypes of what an alcoholic looks like. We are not always easy to spot as we look like everyone else.

Underneath we do share a common bond with the street drinkers but on the surface, we don't look obviously alcoholic. We are users who intentionally imbibe alcohol to change the way we feel about ourselves and our world. For us drinking is more than a take it or leave it recreational and social activity.

A recent poster campaign in hospitals has life-size pictures of normal people with the words 'spot the alcoholic.' The point is that many alcoholics like myself are indistinguishable from anyone else. Our disease is hidden, sometimes even from ourselves.

The myth that you have to be living on a park bench to be an alcoholic is a false one. Many alcoholics live in large houses with mile-long drives. Their drinking is secret, disguised by their respectable and successful lifestyle that just serves to hide their addiction.

This disease is prolific, rampant and often hidden behind smokescreens of respectability and money.

It was this mythology that kept me for many years from knowing that I had this disease.

1.14 Bar Room Vision

When I was nineteen years old, I went for a drink in a bar in Tunbridge Wells. It was a hippie bar and was awash with dope, drink and the occasional live band.

I have a clear memory of walking into that bar, ordering and paying for a small glass of lager, and then looking around the room. In a way that I had not experienced before I received a message from outside of myself. It came in the form of awareness that I was being communicated with by something or someone who I would now identify as God. In essence, the message I was receiving was that 'these people are lost and you are going to do something about it.' I put the drink down without having taken a sip and went out onto the common.

Walking up the path I received an impression, almost a vision, about the future trajectory of my life. I saw that I would not only do something about the people in the bar but that I would be a vicar. I know that I didn't make this up because the next day I was on the train to London and I met the father of a friend of mine. He asked me what I was doing and I told him, but I also said that I was going to become a vicar.

The remarkable thing is that at this point I didn't really believe in God and I didn't even go to Church. In the following months, I tried to fulfil the vision in my own way by signing up for a religious studies course but the studying didn't last long and I just went back to the pub where the vision seemed to die.

1.15 Alcohol on Board

With alcohol on board, I could do crazy and ridiculous things. In my late teens, I rode a motorcycle across a cricket pitch during a company cricket match. I am amazed that I didn't get the sack. Time and again I made a fool of myself by engaging in alcohol-induced behaviour that was out of step with my true character.

With alcohol on board, my alter-ego could take over and all normal sense of reserve and restraint would be thrown to the wind. At the time there was a sense of liberation and freedom as I yielded to its urges but the next day when I sobered up there was usually a sense of remorse as well as damage to be cleared up.

When I was eighteen, I was the passenger in an old Triumph Herald convertible. My best friend was behind the wheel and we had been drinking that day. We had a head-on collision near the bend of a country road. There were no seat belts and I was catapulted through the windscreen, over the bonnet and onto the road. I can still remember it very clearly and what was remarkable is that I just walked away with no real injuries apart from superficial cuts from the glass.

Thankfully, although it was a big impact that wrote off both cars none of us was seriously injured. The first thing that I did when I got home was to go down to the pub for more drinks to celebrate my survival and show off my blood-stained clothes. After that, I went into severe shock and spent several days in bed as my body recovered.

I now see it as a miracle that I was spared serious injury and I honestly think that there must have been angels looking after me that day as there was no human reason for such an escape. I see this as the beginning of alcohol starting to make some serious claims on my life.

1.16 My Right Mind

A friend of mine says that she can tell when her mother has even a small amount of alcohol because she undergoes some sort of personality change.

I recognise this because when I was under the influence of alcohol, even a small amount, I became a different person. Like Jekyll and Hyde alcohol brought about a change in my personality. I was not the same person with a drink inside me and once I was under its power, I was not able to be true to myself.

I used to think it was fun and an adventure into the unknown but now I can see that it was dangerous. At the time the risk and the danger used to carry a sense of excitement but alcohol was just leading me astray and taking my life off course.

Looking back, I can see that from the day I started drinking things started to go wrong. Any willpower that I possessed was removed by alcohol so that the rational Chris might say: 'Chris, it's time to go home,' but the alcohol would overrule and say 'oh, go on have another one.'

Once I got going, I was what drinkers call 'thirsty,' meaning that I had an inexplicable desire and craving for more alcohol. I had little real choice when the compulsion to drink was on me because I was not in my right mind. I couldn't leave it alone.

If I took that one drink in the pub on the way home from work, I found it almost impossible to leave. All my good intentions just evaporated in the atmosphere of drinking. Once I started drinking, I was not in my right mind long before I was drunk.

1.17 The Self-Destruct Button

What it doesn't say on the drink aware label on bottles of booze is that drinking alcohol can cause insanity and death. If alcohol had to go through the same rigorous clinical trials that potential medications do, it would fail to gain approval.

My drinking resulted in a form of arrested development and immaturity that prevented me from growing up. I was at times unpredictable and irrational in a way that I can only put down to drinking. It was almost as if there was some alcoholically induced fifth column at work on the inside who was carrying out acts of sabotage and trying to wreck any positive steps forward that I was trying to take in my life.

At the heart of the illness of alcoholism is the rejection of self and alcohol gave me a self-destruct button which I would press at various points even when I wasn't drinking heavily.

I can still recall the sense of boredom that I felt. Life seemed to have stalled, time seemed to pass so slowly and I didn't know why?

Looking back on it, I can now see that alcohol was already starting to flex its muscles and was preventing me from living the life that I should have been living.

1.18 Temporary Release

Drinking changed the way I felt as it reduced my anxiety and gave me relief from the constant stream of thoughts that were the result of overthinking everything.

Alcohol relativised everything so that nothing seemed that important anymore and I could relax. Drinking gave be a break from life, it gave me time out from every day cares and duties. I felt a massive sense of relief and release when I drank. It was like having a mini-break and I felt that I could breathe and relax in a way that I found difficult without alcohol.

Drink was my way of coping with life and it was great at the time. However, what I realised, later on, was that instead of learning to deal with my feelings and thoughts, I was just stuffing them down and shutting them out with drinking.

The result of this over time was that I became confused and mixed up in my thinking and attitude towards life. I was at sea. I was lost and I was very confused about life.

My response was to retreat to the pub because I knew that in there I could just escape. I was confused about life, but at least alcohol provided some temporary rest bite from this world of confusion that I could not understand.

As I look back, I can see that I was confused, lost and drifting in alcoholic escapism which brought only temporary relief.

1.19 Bottled Up

One of the effects of drinking is that we become much less inhibited and I used to like this. My upbringing has made me very restrained and emotionally uptight so that in my spirit I felt contained and constrained. Alcohol removed my British reserve and I was able to release my inner self in a way that I could not normally do.

Of course, sometimes I would go over the top much to the amusement of my friends, but most of the time I was just letting out aspects of my personality that were bottled up. The real me buried under a heap of emotional repression needed to be released and alcohol provided the pressure release valve. The problem was that I did not know how to express my real self without the chemical assistance of alcohol.

The personality change that I would experience was like flipping a switch. With alcohol I could release my inner self that was normally locked up in a prison of cultural restraint and as I drank the doors would break open and out the real me would come, albeit in an exaggerated form due to the action of the alcohol.

I loved the liberation that came to me when I was drinking as all my cares and self-consciousness just evaporated. I tended to bottle things up and hide my true feelings so alcohol just blew the cork out of my emotional champagne bottle. The release felt great at the time.

1.20 Drinkers Paradise

I remember going on an all-expenses-paid business trip with my boss to visit a company in Ipswich. We got on the train at Liverpool Street Station early in the morning. We went straight to the buffet car where he ordered four large cans of beer and the day continued to follow that pattern of excess until we fell off the return train that evening.

Another time I went on an all-expenses paid day out to the Farnborough Air Show. I was picked up in a limousine and driven to the hospitality tent where I was handed a large gin and tonic and after that, I don't remember much. I never saw a plane and have vague memories of being driven home.

There were the after-work cocktail parties in very smart company reception rooms for visiting clients and these were strictly double gin or double vodka occasions.

There were also the city drinking clubs as well as numerous bars and it was quite acceptable to have a business lunch that stretched late into the afternoon. My boss did most of his business in the marine club with a gin and tonic in hand.

It was all about drinking and it was normalised by the culture of the city at that time. This was the soil in which my drinking habit developed and grew as all normal measures were replaced by large quantities of free drinks.

The city was at that time a drinker's paradise and I willingly partook of its abundance.

1.21 End of the Line

The train home could be a problem after a few drinks. When I was a child, I remember pulling my father out of the first-class compartment and onto the station platform when he'd fallen asleep drunk.

Now I was following in his footsteps. I used to go into blackout when drinking heavily and this meant that I not only had no recall but would also fall unconscious. It wasn't sleeping, it was intoxication and then loss of consciousness.

At Tunbridge Wells, I didn't have anyone to wake me or pull me out, so I remember coming to in the siding of Hastings station at midnight with no way of getting home. I found my way to the Grand Hotel where I was charged a lot of money for a bed.

Very early the next morning the alarm call came through but it was too early to claim my breakfast, so I put on yesterday's clothes, went to the station and caught the train back to London. By the time we arrived at Tunbridge Wells Central, I was triumphantly ensconced in the buffet car with my bacon sandwich and a coffee. My friends who joined me thought this was brilliant and I was unquestionably a drinking hero that day.

There was however nothing heroic about blackout drinking and if I knew what I know about it now, I would not have been laughing.

1.22 Fully Loaded

I remember looking across the desk at my boss who came back loaded from his daily business lunch. He had an amazing thirst for double vodkas and his expense account lunches were all of the liquid variety. On this particular day, he came back 'fully loaded' and just sat there in a comatose state. He may even have been in a blackout.

It was part of a sorry tale of increasing sickness, job loss, lost marriage, homelessness, hospitalisation and death from liver cancer aged fifty. He was not one of the lucky ones. He just could not get recovery and it was heart breaking.

At the time I had little sympathy as I had to cover for him and do his work. In fact, I held resentments against him because of this. However just before he died, I got to speak with him on the phone and I forgave him unconditionally.

At the time I didn't realise that my own drinking career was well underway, but in that environment, it all just seemed to be normal. Drinking was a way of life in the city at that time and no one batted an eyelid unless you fell over or collapsed.

I judged my boss but I was doing much the same thing at a lower level. He had just been doing it for longer and at the time I didn't know anything about alcoholism or have any idea what he was going through at such an advanced level of the disease.

I feel genuine sorrow for him and his family now that I know all that they had to go through. He tried to get recovery and got some measure of sobriety but just couldn't keep it.

1.23 Feeling like a Failure

My self-perception was very distorted as I had a tendency to see myself as a failure. I compared myself with people who were extremely successful. I concluded that I was not very good even though I had a very nice flat in London as well as a good job for someone of my age. This negative self-perception was not based on reality because it had its roots in my childhood and teenage script where I was constantly experiencing failure as a dyslexic in the educational system.

Many like me have also struggled with failure at school and the consequent impact of that on our self-esteem. My sense of being a failure was deeply scripted in me both at school as well as in the family home, so I have had to learn to constantly remind myself that I am not a failure because by the grace of God I have overcome many difficult problems in life, including the drink problem.

This nagging sense of failure made it difficult to acknowledge or celebrate my successes so that when I got a distinction in my master's degree, I just put it down to luck and genuinely told myself that it must have been a fluke or a mistake. I was so scripted in failure that I couldn't embrace the idea that I might succeed at anything. Of course, such feelings inevitably make for more drinking as it becomes the answer to everything.

1.24 Escape Attempts

It would be misleading to give the impression that I never questioned or rebelled against my own drinking habits. I would have periods of reform where I would try to break out of my world of drinking.

In an effort to escape its clutches I joined the territorial army. This failed because when I completed the first six months of training, I joined the Corps of Drums which was inhabited by ex-guardsmen who were all serious drinkers. They used the army reserve as a way of getting out from their normal lives so that they could have some fun and this involved drinking.

I tried some spiritual strategies and attended the Hare Krishna Temple off Oxford Street to see if I could find some answers. I was challenged by their dedication and their way of life that involved a renunciation of Western materialism and a total commitment to their faith. The problem was that not only did they require vegetarianism, but they didn't drink. Eventually, after three months of chanting, I gave way to a few large gin and tonics followed by a ham sandwich and I had to let it all go.

One thing did sort of work and that was something called EST. It was a very expensive series of training sessions and seminars in the Café Royal. I can't explain it but it broke something in me and this enabled me to set out on a different course, which involved being able to move away from the negative influence of the friends with whom I used to drink.

1.25 Mind, Body and Spirit

I attended the exhibition of mind, body and spirit at Earls Court. I was looking for something other than drink and amongst all the weird and wonderful sights, I met some really nice people. I felt a connection and had some form of spiritual experience.

This was followed by a moment of clarity whilst standing on the balcony of my flat as I came to the realisation that there was one answer to all my questions. It was a significant personal revelation and a real breakthrough as many years before I had put these metaphysical ideas in the bin. It was a seed change and I no longer wanted to spend all my time drinking.

Shortly after this I was staying with some friends in Dorset and they obviously thought that I needed some help, so they took me to church. It was a beautiful small country church that had some very famous clear etched glass windows through which the sun was streaming. I remember the strong smell of wood polish but also the thrust of the message that the vicar gave that day.

It was Trinity Sunday and he had the difficult task of trying to explain how in Christian theology God is one, but also three persons as revealed in the Father, the Son and the Holy Spirit. I followed his message as far as I could, perhaps just for a few minutes until I zoned out, but I got the information that I needed. What his message did was to bring the idea of God back into my thinking.

Although I didn't realise the significance of this at the time, what happened to me that day, was that I started to think about God, and I suspect that this was when I started to reach outside of myself towards a higher power in my search for answers to all my mental confusion about life.

It wasn't long after that visit that I found myself in a church where I was helped to come to a living faith in God. It didn't stop me from drinking but it did provide a pathway out of some of my confusion and mental chaos that had been exacerbated by alcohol.

1.26 Deception and Denial

I would like to give an account of how I was miraculously delivered out of my life of debauchery and wafted into a new level of existence where my now spiritualised life became one of continuous progress into the Himalayas of spiritual experience. The sad truth is that it took me the next thirty years before I could begin to truly let go of alcohol and get released from its effect on my life.

My journey was not to be a straightforward ascent but a long and winding path with many obstacles and setbacks along its circuitous route.

As I embarked on a new journey into the world of religion, I had no idea what I was getting into or the trouble that I was going to have because of my previous marriage to the bottle. I thought that I could just walk out and leave my old life of drinking behind me, but I never bargained for the fact that I had only separated and not divorced. The was no decree absolute and no legal separation from my previous relationship with alcohol. Even though I didn't realise it at the time I had not broken the unseen cords that bound me.

Once established as a habit, destructive drinking protects itself like a virus that mutates into different strains and forms. In its early stages it hides, it lies and tells you that it's not a problem.

Alcoholism is patient, lying low and seemingly dormant for many years, just waiting for an opportune time. At times you can think it's gone away and that your drinking problem has disappeared. Denial moves in to mask the truth, whilst the illness progresses unchallenged until like a tarantula it bursts out of hiding showing its full force and deadly control over its unwitting victim.

As I set out on the spiritual path, I thought that my drinking days were behind me and that I was now free to get on and live the life that I was meant to live. I was deluded and naïve to think that alcohol would let go of me that easily.

1.27 New York City Blues

When I was working in the city, I won a business scholarship to go to the United States to get the feel of some of the major business houses in New York. We flew business class and stayed in the Plaza hotel enjoying the gastronomic delights of New York's finest restaurants and of course we drank a lot of alcohol. I met some amazing people including the people who managed the twin towers of the world trade centre.

Finding myself with some free time, I walked up the side of central park to the Frick Gallery where for just a dollar you could see the Frick family art collection. I walked into one of the rooms and there was a huge picture of St Francis of Assisi in the desert by Giovani Bernini. Francis was pictured outside his cave with his prayer stool and the scriptures open in front of him. The painting is called the ecstasy of St Francis and I know why, because when I looked at the picture, I burst into tears, as it connected with me in a most profound way.

As I looked up at that painting, I knew that I was being called out of my life in business and into the sort of life represented by St Francis. It was totally unexpected, but after that, I just wanted to go home.

The whole trip was rather like the temptation of Christ in the wilderness as I was being shown the kingdom of this world with all of its power and the wealth behind it.

But I also had an awakening to my calling which was out of that business world and into a new life as a vicar.

1.28 The Rector

I was recently thanked for a meeting that I held for a small group of alcoholics at the local detoxification centre where I help as a voluntary chaplain. One of the things that they thanked me for was not preaching to them. I think what they meant was that I had been honest and not tried to lecture or speak down to them.

I understand where my friends were coming from but I don't despise preaching because for me it has really helped me to understand God, myself and the world. I needed information and it was a preacher who provided me with it. He was the Rector of the Church next to where I worked in the city. It had an impressive congregation with about five hundred people showing up for the lunch hour talks.

On my first visit, the preacher caught me at the door and invited me for a cup of tea and a doughnut. I never got the doughnut but he did explain his message which I gladly received. Significantly I felt that this man really believed what he was telling me and I was struck by his sincerity. I had never encountered that sort of conviction and spiritual authority before.

From then on, I just went to everything he did and spent as much time in his company as I could. It wasn't hero worship it was just that he had the message that I needed. What he said was honest, straight and he spoke my language. It wasn't the usual series of religious platitudes that I had been used to in the school chapel.

It was an amazing time in my life and it took my attention right off drinking. I had found a different spirit and it was a better one.

1.29 Fighting Drink

As I left the drinking scene and replaced my drinking friends with other people who were focussing on their spiritual lives it was a lot easier not to drink. Initially, I had a big fight on my hands as my desire to drink waged war with my newfound desire not to take a drink. I was internally conflicted and the way I got through it was to replace drinking activities with non-drinking activities, which diverted my thinking and my energy away from the drink.

Instead of going to the pub after work, I volunteered at a youth club in the East End. It was a non-drinking environment and it kept me occupied so that I wasn't focused on the absence of alcohol. I got involved in small group studies and volunteered for various practical duties within a congregation. At lunchtimes I would visit churches where they had coffee and tea rather than the bars and pubs that had been my usual watering holes.

It was a massive fight to break free from the pattern of habitual drinking that I had been involved in for quite a few years. What I didn't realise at the time was that this was just the start of a long-running battle with alcohol. I had no idea what a formidable enemy I was up against.

The former England Cricketer and African missionary C.T.Studd used to say that the young recruits who came to him in Africa were trying to kill elephants with pea shooters. They didn't have the power or the program to deal with the elephantine spiritual force of darkness that was coming against them.

I didn't realise how serious my condition was or how deeply rooted my obsession with drinking had become. I didn't have a clue what a fight I was going to have with this enemy of my soul and all I had to fight it with at the time was a pea shooter.

1.30 New Identity

As I grew in my new identity the sub-cultural boundaries of the faith community were made very clear.

Drinking was fine in moderation but drunkenness was unacceptable on any occasion.

Although my drinking had been down-graded to the occasional drink I was still smoking a lot. I was cross-addicted and so my addiction just jumped to cigarettes which I smoked with a vengeance.

Again, in my newfound social world smoking was frowned upon if not regarded as sinful. I tried many things to kick the habit including flushing the cigarettes down the toilet on numerous occasions. In the end, I was desperate and went into the Church to pray. I met a person who saw my distress and prayed with me. I have never smoked since.

I wish it had been like that with my drinking and that I could have stopped forever at that time. It was 1982 and I was making progress in life without being drunk and without cigarettes. Contrary to popular opinion life without these things wasn't boring, in fact, it was a lot better than the mess that I had been in before.

My old identity started to fade as I began to embrace the lifestyle of a young professional conservative evangelical complete with leather zipped pocket Bible, Filofax and Barbour.

1.31 Wrestling for Control

Most of the time I managed to keep it together in terms of my behaviour and I knew that I had God in my life in a way that I had not before, but from time to time I would have a slip and drink too much.

On average these slips took place every three or four months but they were embarrassing and I felt bad that I couldn't live an absolutely consistent Christian life.

These slips were all alcohol-related and were the result of me being in situations where for some reason I was not able to control my drinking. I was alright as long as I didn't take a drink but after a few beers with my colleagues, I would get the taste and want to keep going.

I wasn't staggering around afterwards but I knew in myself that I had drunk too much and I would always feel that I had let both God and myself down. I would vow to be more careful in the future and it could be many months before this would happen again, but it always did, and I couldn't understand why. I felt bad and embarrassed but I could never figure out how it had happened.

I can now see that I just clicked straight back into the pattern of drinking that was already established in my body and brain. After the first drink, I had little choice in the matter, it was almost automatic.

This would be my pattern for the next twenty-five years as I wrestled with the urge to drink and the desire not to.

February

2.1 Spiritual Experience

I was blessed with a vivid spiritual experience in my earliest days in the church. I went to a lunchtime service and there was a reading from the book of the prophet Isaiah where he is commissioned to take the message out to people who will be ever hearing but never listening.

Not only did it eventually come true for me but it spoke to me in the deepest places of my being. It was a real connection with my higher power that is my God. It was as if I was being spoken to personally and although I didn't hear an actual voice it moved me deep within. I think this spiritual experience was part of my call to the priesthood, but at the time I didn't realise it.

This and other spiritual experiences did not stop me from drinking. The church is not tea-total and therefore it was not obvious to me that I should stop drinking entirely. I hear of people who do have spiritual experiences that result in them stopping drinking immediately but I wasn't one of them. There was no thunderbolt from heaven or flash of lightning and I certainly never picked up the idea that my drinking was in conflict with my faith.

Nobody amongst my new circle of spiritually-minded friends had any experience of alcoholism which meant that they couldn't give me a steer. So, on the one hand, I was having powerful spiritual experiences, and on the other, trips to the pub.

2.2 Lack of Information

What I didn't possess back then was any knowledge about my true condition. I had no understanding about how serious my addiction was although I do remember walking back to my flat one day and feeling like I was just hanging from a wall by my fingernails. I was twenty-three years old and without knowing it, I was already an alcoholic.

Most of the time I didn't drink and I was drinking very little apart from the occasional slip. I just didn't know that I had gone so far with my drinking that it was never going to be possible for me to drink normally again. I had no information and because after a short period of struggle, I didn't seem to have an obvious problem on a day-to-day basis, I didn't seek out any further help. I thought that by not drinking my body and mind would just do a factory reset.

I didn't know that even with a living faith and God in my life I was going to face a lifetime of confusion and defeat with alcohol. I thought that my days of heavy drinking were behind me and that in my new life as a Christian I would be able to just walk away from this problem. What I didn't know then was that true alcoholism is an incurable and progressive illness that without treatment usually ends in death. I just didn't have this information and neither had I met anyone who had.

I had no idea that I had crossed some invisible boundary, a point of no return with my drinking.

2.3 The Wine Bar

The bottles of German beer and toasted cheese sandwiches at the Jamaica wine bar in St Michael's Alley,

Cornhill were the regular feature of my broker's lunch and although the drink did affect me, I was far from drunk.

My boss used to take us for a proper business lunch at the George and Vulture or Simpsons, where we used to eat whitebait followed by steak pie or some other form of traditional English food. This would be accompanied by top-quality claret and followed by port. It was difficult to function after these lunches and my breath used to smell like a jet engine but it was great fun and I have some brilliant memories of these occasions.

My boss was an immense character who in his retirement bought a chateau in France and became a devout Roman Catholic. Looking back, I can see that this was pretty epic drinking in relation to today's standards which measures units and the like. However, at the time it was considered perfectly reasonable and my conscience was not too troubled by it.

We worked hard, we were good at what we did, and we made the company millions of pounds a year, so the occasional serious lunch didn't seem wrong or out of place in the scheme of things.

Ironically the first recovery meeting I ever attended some twenty-five years later was held in the vestry of St Michaels Cornhill right opposite the Jamaica wine bar.

2.4 Prison Fellowship

I am always interested in how people come into our lives at just the right time. One of the people who came into my life at the right time was a former presidential lawyer, Charles Colson. I heard him speak twice and both times I was deeply touched by God. He was working through his prison fellowship organisation for reconciliation and peace between IRA and Unionist prisoners in the H Block prisons in Northern Ireland.

Through the Watergate scandal, he had found himself going from the president's office to the federal penitentiary. It was a mighty fall for a great man but it had opened the door for his life's work in prison reform and as an advocate for prisoners and their families. He said that no one's life was wasted when it was given to God and at the time, I felt that I was wasting my life.

I wanted to do something for God that would have an impact but I didn't know what. I think this was all part of my calling but it would take some time for it to be realised. I guess it is still unravelling as I find myself increasingly working with other alcoholics and addicts.

My fall from grace was not public or dramatic but eventually when alcohol brought me to my knees it opened up a new life where I could be of use to others. I will never be able to do even a fraction of what Colson did for suffering prisoners, many of whom were incarcerated because of drugs and alcohol, but his life showed me that God can take our biggest humiliations and turn them around so that they become our greatest assets.

2.5 Keswick

Many people have been touched by God in Keswick at the annual Keswick Convention. The originator of the Oxford Group that was behind the twelve-step programs of recovery was himself radically touched by God at Keswick. I was taken to the Keswick Convention and whilst I was there, I had a profound experience of God. Most notably during a sermon by the Reverend Eric Alexander who was a preacher from Glasgow.

He spoke about the human wreckage that was being washed up on his church doorstep every day. There was an epidemic of drug and alcohol misuse in Glasgow at the time and he was in the middle of it. His exhortation was that we should devote ourselves to prayer and the ministry of the word in order to find God's direction and purpose for us in these situations of desperate need.

I sensed deeply that his message had my name on it and a strange thing happened to me afterwards. I could not speak for about twenty minutes as I was rendered completely dumb. I guess you could call it dumbstruck. God had spoken to me and I was rendered speechless.

That time at Keswick was significant and supernatural. It was my calling to prayer and the ministry of the word but the picture in my mind's eye as he spoke was also significant as I imagined the drug addicts and alcoholics at the door of his church who were coming to him for help.

It is no coincidence that over the years as a priest, I have found that God brings alcoholics and drug addicts to my door in different ways and at different times.

2.6 Drink Free Environment

As a result of my newfound faith, I met my future wife, not in a bar or a club, but on a church-sponsored New Year's retreat at a country house in Surrey. We followed the church rules by living apart until married and we had a smart city wedding.

Before our marriage, we had responded to a call for help from the vicar of St Johns Church Hoxton which had a very magnificent but at the time a rather dilapidated Hawksmore style building. We ran a pathfinder youth group for five children in this inner-city parish and I helped the vicar with leading services. He had been a missionary in South America and had developed a preaching course so he went through it with me and taught me to preach.

This was a drink-free environment and it suited me well because there was no temptation to indulge and it was while I was helping the vicar with church services that my vision about becoming a priest was brought back to life.

Looking back on those days, I can now see that although I wasn't drinking, I was struggling with the emotional issues that come with being a 'dry drunk.' A dry drunk is an alcoholic who is not drinking but is not getting help with the roots of the underlying addiction which is still there below the surface of things.

Whilst I was putting on a good show outwardly my real mental state was far from peaceful as I was suffering from what I now understand as untreated alcoholism.

2.7 Internal Struggles

Although I didn't really understand it at the time, I was struggling with the emotional health issues that would affect any addict who has come out of substance abuse. At times, particularly at work , I experienced very high levels of fear and anxiety which were almost unbearable.

I found early married life quite difficult to adjust to because I had spent the years when I should have been developing as a person just drinking in the pub. I found it difficult to live with myself let alone my beautiful young wife.

I would spend a lot of my free time on my own just reading as a way of coping. This was not good for our new marriage relationship and one day, my wife said to me in frustration, 'I think I married a book.' It was just my way of escaping and trying to deal with the volcano of untreated alcoholic magma boiling away within me.

I didn't know what was going on and I certainly had no clue that it had anything to do with alcohol. This was a long time before the awareness that there is today about mental health and addiction issues, so I just sat it out and got on with life the best I could.

2.8 Significant Others

At some key turning points in my life, people have been sent across my path who perhaps unknown to them have been used as catalysts for significant and positive change.

My senior manager at work was one such person who helped me to realise that I needed to change the whole course of my life. He was a very dynamic lawyer who was working in the company to gain the experience that he would later use in the establishment of a successful law practice.

At my annual review, he got me to talk about my voluntary work with the inner-city church youth group at St John's church in Hoxton. I chatted away enthusiastically about what I was doing and my hopes for the group while he just listened. Then he got me to talk about my work in the company. At end of the conversation, he asked me to compare the enthusiastic way that I had spoken about my voluntary work compared with the rather lacklustre way I had spoken about my paid job.

He helped me to see where my heart was and that it wasn't in the work that I had been doing up to this time.

I am so thankful to that man who was brought across my path just at the right time. It wasn't to be too long before I left that business to enter into my true life's work as a priest in the Church of England.

We just don't know or realise the difference that we can make in other people's lives.

2.9 Emotional Health

I swapped out my city job for a Church one after some serious soul searching about the fact that I had to take a massive drop in income. I was already in the system for ordination training having been provisionally accepted as an ordinand in the Church of England.

I worked as an assistant in a church for two years and then went to Theological College. Being away from the city drinking and any sort of drinking culture made me feel that my life had moved on and that my drinking life was now all behind me.

I was careful around drink and drinking occasions and I can't remember getting drunk at all over that time. I would have said that my problem drinking was in the past and so it stayed right through my college days and into my first post as a priest. As one of my friends would say alcohol was just out of sight in the backroom doing press-ups.

There were some clues that all was not well within me. I could behave irrationally and impulsively which worried me and my head was not always in a good place, but I was too scared to talk with anyone and I didn't really recognise that I had unresolved emotional problems.

We studied pastoral counselling but what I needed was someone to counsel me and to work through my issues before going into the priesthood.

2.10 Spiritual Non-conformist

One of my great grandfathers was a Wesleyan Methodist missionary who died of black water fever on the mission field in East Africa. His non-conformist approach to religion was in my blood and this surfaced as I found the religious aspects of my theological college very difficult to accept.

I hit up against the difference between spirituality and religion. I had come from a form of spirituality that regarded the place of encounter with God as being internal and personal as well as out there in life rather than locked up in some chapel or religious institution. Chapel services, priests, robes, liturgies, candles, and all the other paraphernalia of religion held little interest for me.

Unlike my personal spiritual experience, the religious tradition that I was being asked to embrace felt very unnatural. My faith was internal as well as out there in the market place but the religious side of things left me cold.

I felt that I was continually being pressed to become something that I was not. The more pressure that I was put under to be religious the more I found myself resisting. My non-conformist background kicked in and I found it difficult to conform to the formal religious expressions of faith that were being forced upon me.

I knew that I'd been called to be a priest just not a religious one.

2.11 What and How

At theological college a friend read me a piece from a book. It was all about the difference between the what and the how of belief.

It made the point that we were all getting very good at the what of our faith in terms of what we believed but the problem facing us was how were we going to live it? We subscribed to the tenets of our faith and to the way of life that was being prescribed, the problem was that we just couldn't live up to it.

I was acutely aware of this given my underlying alcohol problem and some of my friends had similar struggles but in other areas of their lives. Some were having problems with sex, others were having problems with their marriages, their money or their sexual identity.

These problems were never addressed and we all had to pretend that we were all okay. If we had admitted that we were struggling or transgressing in these areas we would probably have been ejected from the training process, so we all just kept quiet.

There was an unreality and disconnect about the training process as it was all about gaining more intellectual knowledge at the expense of a real experience of God and his work in our lives.

As I found out more and more about what the scriptures said, I found myself less and less able to do it. I knew a lot about my faith in terms of beliefs, but little about how to live it in practice, let alone showing others how to do it.

2.12 Two Spirits

When I was at theological college one of the African students went to the barbers and sat next to a man in the queue who was drinking a can of beer. My African friend said to the man with the beer, 'I know a better spirit than that one.' The man was rather taken aback but a friendly conversation ensued.

I was aware that through my faith I had received a new spirit and I could sense the movement and work of that spirit within me. I believe it was the Spirit of God working inside me in some mystical way that is beyond the purely physical realm.

However, there was at the same time another spirit that was still exercising power and influence in my life even though I didn't realise it. Most of the time it was hidden, fairly well behaved and under control but it was just lying low and keeping its head down until an opportune time.

The doorway for its entry was still ajar and I had no idea that this spirit would take advantage of every opportunity that I was to give it by not totally closing the door on it. All I had to do to allow it in was to take a drink. I didn't understand this at the time, after all, what's wrong with a drink?

Eventually, I would come to the point of closing the door on it completely, but only after it had done a lot of damage.

I wish I had known this at the time but I didn't know what was going on and I could not see the situation as clearly as I can now. The Spirit of God would not share my body with any other spirits, they would have to go.

2.13 Power and Powerlessness

I thought that I had the power that I needed to conquer any problem that I might have with drinking. I believed that the combination of my own willpower and my faith in God would be able to see me through. What I failed to realise was the power and grip that alcohol already had on my life. Deep down it had hold of me and I was still holding onto it.

It was like an illicit love affair that I was not willing to let go of. My soul was still tied to alcohol at the deepest level. No matter how much I tried I just could not release its grip on me. I had to learn that I was going to continually fail to get free as long as I thought that I could gain power over alcohol by means of my own will, determination, and strength.

What I eventually discovered was a paradox. As long as I held onto the idea that I had the power over alcohol I could not overcome it, but once I admitted that I was powerless I was able to access a higher power, which was to bring me deliverance. My understanding of that higher power is that it is the power of God and it was this power that eventually broke the chains of alcohol in my heart, my mind, and my body.

However, I had to be willing and at that point in my life, I was not really willing to let go as I was bound far more tightly to alcohol than I could ever have imagined at the time.

2.14 Only One Man

Only one man recognised my struggle at this time. In fact, he realised the gravity of my potential problem with drink years before I did. I thank God for this man because he prepared me for what was to come and gave me the information that would ultimately save my life.

He was a Baptist minister and a non-drinker for the first fifty years of his life, having only taken up drinking later in life. He had found himself increasingly dependent on alcohol and having recovered he was intentionally putting information into me so that if I did give way again to problem drinking, I would know what to do.

Deep down I sort of knew that he had my number, and oddly because of that I didn't go and see him anymore, it was too uncomfortable.

He was the only person who ever levelled with me about their drinking and he was a minister, which meant that I wasn't the only one in Christian ministry operating with this weakness.

I've still got a signed copy of his own daily reading book that he gave to me during that time. I value it very much because he died before I found release from my drinking, so I wasn't able to celebrate my recovery with him.

2.15 The Information

As a curate, that is a trainee priest in the Church of England, I lived next to a church hall where a rather strange meeting took place every Wednesday night. I used to watch people going into these meetings and I was intrigued especially one night when there was a highly visible altercation.

I think it was partly because of the information that was being planted in my mind by my Baptist friend as well as at a more mysteriously level I had experienced a sense of being drawn to attend these meetings.

One night I plucked up the courage and said to my wife that I was going to see what these people were doing. It was an open meeting and I was warmly welcomed. One of the men gave me a daily reflections book which he signed with his name and phone number.

I remember coming home and saying to my wife 'I think I am one of those people.' In my subconscious, I had identified with their experiences but my conscious mind took many more years to catch up. From time to time, I would occasionally pick up the daily reflections book and read it.

However, I wasn't ready to seek any sort of recovery because I didn't know how serious my problem was at that time. It didn't look like I had a drinking problem because I didn't drink much.

But when alcohol eventually proved its point, I knew that there were people who spoke my language, understood what I was experiencing and could help me.

2.16 A Bit More Information

During my time as a trainee priest, I got friendly with a man in our church who had been a full-on alcoholic but had recovered through Alcoholics Anonymous and then joined the church.

He and his wife told me about his out-of-control drinking and the way he had been completely given over to his alcoholism. He had fallen asleep in people's gardens and generally lost control of his drinking having become a continual consumer of alcohol. I was fascinated by his story as I identified so much with it.

I had no idea at the time that I was an alcoholic just like him but I was gripped by his story and I liked to spend time with him and his wife. I think that deep in my heart I knew that he had found something that I wanted.

Although I wasn't drinking, I was not free from alcoholism and I had met someone who had found a way out of this hopeless addiction.

He had no idea why I should be so interested in his story and eventually he didn't want to talk about it anymore.

He broke free from alcoholic drinking but as I think back, I can see that he was still manifesting signs of alcoholism even though it was kept at bay by his church life.

2.17 No Not Yet

My resistance to the idea that I might one day have to address my drinking was weakened over time. I moved from an absolute no, with the attitude that I will never give up drinking, towards a position of not yet.

I wasn't willing or able to contemplate a life without the drink and I could not at this stage of my life imagine giving up alcohol forever.

I not only drank for fun but I was a user in the sense that I was self-medicating with drink, and it served a purpose in keeping the lid on some deeply rooted pain in my life.

I didn't understand it or know it at a conscious level but I was carrying a lot of pain and shame from my past that had not been processed. The drink served a purpose for me as it anesthetised me from feeling the pain of my abusive family life, abuse at school and dyslexia, as well as many other wounds that I had picked up along the way.

At this stage of my life alcohol still worked for me in dulling the pain and giving me a break from my emotional and mental noise. Of course, what the alcohol was doing was providing temporary respite with short-term relief and release from unwanted feelings.

For many years I shut down my feelings so that it was impossible for me to cry or even to know what I was feeling.

Slowly but steadily my consumption increased as I needed more alcohol to do the same job. There would be times of trying to cut back followed by periods of excess.

In my heart of hearts, I knew that one day it would have to come to an end and that I would have to give in to what I believe is the will of God for my life. That is no alcohol at all.

2.18 The Priest and the Bottle

My drinking crept back slowly over a period of fourteen years. Like the tide at Lindisfarne, it came in stealthily and without obvious waves. I had no idea at this juncture that it would in time overwhelm me.

I had no intention of becoming a drunken priest and I was not going to give in to alcohol, but the tide would prove to be far stronger than I could ever have imagined.

Although I had no intention surrendering to the bottle, alcohol was never far away. When I was installed as the Priest-in-Charge of St Mary's Church there were no facilities in the church building at the time so the bishop and clergy had to robe up in the saloon bar of the pub. How cool was that?

A well-known London hotelier provided top-quality champagne on ice in the vestry and so my ministry as a parish priest began.

My theological training was of little initial value but all the years I had spent drinking in the city meant that I knew what to do in the pub. People welcomed me and I have always enjoyed humorous banter and a good reception.

The people in the pub loved the fact that their Rector liked a drink and even now I am always bought a drink when I go in there. They offer me a Guinness because they would love to see me back on it.

I suppose that in a strange sort of way my drinking used to give them all permission to imbibe.

2.19 Ordinary Time

In the Church calendar, there is a gap between Trinity Sunday and Advent which is called ordinary time. Basically, not a lot happens between Trinity Sunday in June and Advent at beginning of December.

The first ten years of my ministry in the parish was like ordinary time as far as my drinking went, not a lot happened. There was still the odd slip or scrape but on the whole, drink was not a feature of these years.

I had a young family and my work took over my life. I was absolutely determined to make the church a success and I poured my whole self into its development. Instead of drink being my number one priority, work took over.

The needs of my wife and the children were subordinated to this great obsession with making these dry bones live so my addiction jumped ship from alcohol to work. I was always trying some new initiative to promote the growth and life of the congregation. I am sure we did some good but our efforts failed to secure the results that we or the people who had employed us were looking for. Selling God in a materialist culture was far harder than I had ever imagined.

At the beginning of the new millennium, I took up running as a way of doing something other than Church. I had been a good runner at school and my neighbour was a keen member of the local running club. I joined and ran numerous half-marathons as well as three London Marathons.

The running club was a 'Hash House Harriers' club so that involved drinking. The club motto was 'the running club with a drinking problem' and this was true. The evening training sessions were followed by drinking sessions in the pub that undid all the good work achieved on the run.

So, even in ordinary time alcohol was able to take a little more ground in my life under the guise of work and healthy exercise.

2.20 Not Enough

After nearly ten years as a parish priest, my wife got cancer and at the same time, I was debilitated with a severe kidney infection. At one point we thought that we might lose the battle with cancer and it was a difficult time. I was in a lot of pain and my medical problems didn't get sorted out until I was referred to a Harley Street consultant through St Luke's Hospital for the Clergy.

At this time, I received a most devastating letter of complaint and personal criticism of my ministry from one of the disgruntled members of the Church. It was bad timing and it brought me very low. As a result of this, I became angry with God and with the Church. I was resentful because I felt that I had been let down by God and conned by the Church. This was a bad situation on every front.

When the consultant urologist asked me how much I drank, I replied 'not enough', and after that, I intentionally bought a bottle of wine and drank it whilst sitting in front of the log fire in my sitting room. It made me feel better about things, but the resentment that I'd picked up against God and the Church went deep down into my heart.

I was angry with God and with this person who was giving me abuse when all I was trying to do was the best that I could to serve God in a very challenging set of circumstances.

This resentment was the catalyst for my ultimate descent into renewed serious drinking.

2.21 The Loose Cannons

I was approached by a friend at the local rugby club and asked if I would be willing to teach some of the young people who were interested in playing rock music.

I have played the drums from about the age of eleven when my cousin got me going with a pair of sticks, a practice pad and a Jack Parnell rudiments of drumming book. At school, I played in the orchestra, marching band, the jazz band and later in some rock bands. My school had a history of producing rock bands including the band 'Keene.'

I wasn't one of the superstars but I could play the drums and after a lot of persuading, I took my drums to the club and alongside a bass player and guitarist we tried to teach the youth to play in a band. All of them eventually dropped out but we ended up jamming and formed a band which we called the Loose Cannons.

We played together for five years as a local function band mostly playing in pubs. We even did a biker's gig in the Cathedral and got to play Hendrix in the nave. Of course, like most rock bands, the gigs and the rehearsals all involved drinking. I could play better after a few drinks because I felt more relaxed behind the kit. It never seemed the same when we were playing sober and I think we all played better when we were drinking, at least we thought so.

The only downside was that it did involve being in pubs and clubs where there was a lot of drinking going on and it was difficult not to participate.

2.22 Death of a Vision

My vision of a thriving church with young families and a vibrant spiritual community gradually began to die as I worked in the real world of early 21st century British culture. Sunday shopping, children's sports and general apathy toward anything other than material pursuits made running a church difficult and discouraging.

When I first entered the church, I belonged to a congregation where over a thousand people would gather for Sunday evening and mid-week services. In such an environment it was easy to see that this was a good and impressive thing. But in a cold, smelly and uninspiring village hall on a Sunday morning with eighteen people, some challenging acoustics and a floor sticky with last night's beer, it was a different matter altogether.

Some people abandoned me to seek more promising and successful looking churches in the towns and others just drifted away. My loyal band of followers stuck with me, as did the people in the community who would come for christenings, weddings or funerals.

My vision for revival and renewal slowly began to wither and die. More sickness at home meant that I was in charge of domestic arrangements for the family and for a time assumed the role of carer for my wife who struggled with post-viral fatigue syndrome.

Most of the time I rose above these circumstances but as time went on the bottle began to speak to me once more.

2.23 The Dinner Party

Some people in the church invited me and my wife over to their house for dinner. I was really enjoying myself, not because of the drink, but because of the friendship and the laughter.

Suddenly the conversation changed and I was asked if I would take their daughter's wedding. It wasn't a bad thing that they wanted from me and I was happy to oblige.

They had invited me over because they wanted to get me to do something for them. I am sure this wasn't the first time this had happened but I remember feeling very alone after that and realising that in any position of power, however limited, people often just want you for what they can get out of you. It hit me that being the priest affected, skewed and coloured all normal relationships with people.

Thankfully in recovery, I have had the opposite experience as people have accepted me and loved me as I am and for who I am, and not for what they can get out of me.

Most of them don't even know that I am a priest and therefore the relationships are not coloured in the same way as they are in the parish context.

2.24 Lambs to the Slaughter

I was angry and resentful towards the Church of England as I felt that I had been conned and used. It felt that I had been led like a lamb to the slaughter, cannon fodder that had been sent out into the front-line trenches to be blown to pieces. I had no idea about the reality of being a vicar in a small parish church. I had come from big churches that were growing and where many young people were attending and participating.

My expectations were high and I thought that I could make a success of the place even though one of my colleagues at the time described the parish as 'the graveyard of ambition.' I saw it all through rose-coloured spectacles but there was a mine-field of local and family politics as well as what people can't see, which is the spiritual pressure of being a priest in a rural community.

It is not really explicable if you have not experienced it but just being there and living in the Rectory gave me a constant sense of being observed, and I felt that I was on duty the whole time. I felt that I always should be doing something to justify my being there, and I found it difficult to relax, which is why the drink was so useful.

Then there was the feedback on my performance which would usually be introduced with the words 'people are saying.' No one would say who these people were and they rarely identified themselves or came forward to share their views with me directly.

Their critique of my ministry always came indirectly and I was never really sure what the issues were so it was difficult to respond. I wonder now if the 'people who were saying' were the same people who were being nice to my face and even flattering me, but undermining me behind my back?

Having started with such a high vision and expectation of priestly life in a community this was developing into a tough assignment and I began to struggle.

2.25 Obsessive Disposition

My faith started to undergo a transition as I became disillusioned with the endless promises of turnarounds in the Church. By this, I mean the continual stream of people and programs that promised revival and growth. I would attend conferences where I would hear all these remarkable stories of what God was doing, which was great, but why wasn't it happening here? Their upbeat message contrasted with my own lived experience of struggle and few apparent results for my labours in the field of faith.

Spiritually I felt like I was in a goldfish bowl, just swimming round and round but not getting anywhere. I wanted to grow in my faith and to know God better but what I was doing wasn't working. I was stuck.

It was a great relief when one summer I went to a seminar where I had the opportunity to talk it all through with an academic theologian who suggested that I study at his university faculty. He thought that I needed to process my experience of faith and ministry and he was right. I jumped at the opportunity.

Within six weeks of that conversation, I found myself on a Master's degree course studying theology. It was a lifesaver, absolutely brilliant and I loved it. It was just what I needed because it enabled me to reflect and to think about what I had been doing in my life and ministry up to this point.

My studies also kept me away from drinking because I had a new focus and I was enjoying what I was learning as it was life-giving.

I put my obsessive disposition to work and was awarded a distinction along with the offer of a place to study for a research degree.

2.26 Choose Life

Walking across Charing Cross bridge one bright sunny morning on the way to the university I was hit by an overwhelming desire to go for a drink. It was only nine in the morning but this thought was very dominant and persistent. I can now see that this was a fork in the road of my life and a turning point.

In my mind's eye, I could see two destinies. I knew that if I obeyed the urge to take a drink I would be dropping out of my life and heading for the street. I had the impression that if I took that road there was no coming back. It would have been going out into the night. I would have been joining the outcasts who roam our towns and cities.

It was a frightening experience as I came face to face with the raw and destructive power of my obsession with alcohol. This really shocked me and although I didn't realise it at the time, it was just another insight into how much of a problem I had. Thankfully I carried on walking, went to a lecture and continued to finish my studies at the university.

That day I chose life and although things seemed to get worse, I think the decision I made that day was the beginning of my recovery and the start of my escape from the grip of addiction.

2.27 Old Habits Die Hard

My drinking was habitual. It was based around a web of habits that had been reinforced through my teenage years. When I drank, I would unconsciously click back into one of these patterns of drinking. It was an automatic setting in my brain that just switched on without me realising it. I would find myself operating on automatic pilot and without thinking would go off on a binge.

At the time I didn't realise that this was happening as I wasn't really conscious of what I was doing. I can now see that I was just following one of a number of pre-set drinking programs that had become hard-wired in my brain.

I still experience moments when these old patterns are triggered by some event or thought, but of course, I no longer act on them. I take note but I have the power of choice, and I no longer act out of these old programs.

2.28 Losing Control

A three-month sabbatical had given me the time and the space to write my Master's thesis, but this time out from the parish also brought my drink problem to a head. My drinking just seemed to accelerate once I was free from the daily obligations of my work. I enjoyed the freedom of being a normal person for a few months without the sense of responsibility and duty that comes with the priesthood.

The problem was that I enjoyed the freedom too much so that when I had to return to my parish work, I was struggling. It was hard to go back and my drinking had gone up more than a few notches over my summer of study and recreation.

I had also finished my Masters so I had nothing to focus on or to work towards. For the following eight months my drinking was back to what it had been in my early twenties. I had somehow just clicked back into my old patterns from over thirty years before.

I managed to make it through Christmas and into the New Year but by the early spring, I knew I was in deep trouble. I needed a red emergency escape button but there wasn't one. I had hit rock bottom.

A few years before I'd seen a counsellor. I called her and left a message which said 'I'm in real trouble, can you help me?' She saw me immediately and from then on, I was in her counselling office every week for over eighteen months.

Her intervention saved me from losing everything, maybe even my life.

2.29 Slow Train Coming

It took me a long time in counselling to get to the point where I could start to let go and to let the light in. I'd always been very secretive and closed to everyone so it was difficult to share.

My counsellor was very patient and she had a sense of how far she could go with me each week. I now realise that by calling for help I had let go and let God.

That phone call was so significant as I had reached out for help. I had admitted that I could not control this thing that was driving me to drink. I couldn't do it by myself anymore. I could no longer ignore it or stuff it down with booze. I had to reach out to another human being for help and as I did so I found the hand of God through that person.

It took a long time as a lifetime of denial had to be dismantled and ways forward had to be found. My whole life had been built on sand and so with the help of the counsellor I had to start rebuilding from the ground up.

As a builder friend of mine used to say 'the money is in the ground.' In other words, no matter how splendid the building looks if you build it on poor or cheap foundations, it will eventually crack and fall down. That is exactly what had happened to me.

March

3.1 The Roots

Counselling revealed the roots of my drinking. The lid came off and out came all sorts of things that I had buried. I had built my life on a landfill site as I had buried so much of my past, particularly my childhood. I covered it over and just carried on. I thought that I could just ignore it and pretend that it wasn't there. But now the covering was being removed and what was being revealed was a mass of rubbish from the past that had never been sorted or processed. As long as it remained in this state it was polluting and poisoning my life.

In the counselling room, piece by piece these decomposing remains from my early life started being excavated. In fact, what I came to realise was that my past was not a waste heap but a valuable resource that was being processed and recycled. It would go on to be used to help others, particularly those who were seeking to escape from the mess of drinking. Instead of covering up the past by drinking on it, I was now letting it see the light of day so that everything of value could be extracted and used for good.

Like nettles, the roots were difficult to expose and deal with but the time had come and I knew that I needed to do the work if I was to live free of my past and the underground pressures that it exerted especially in the need to drink.

3.2 Firm Foundations

I have been driving past a sink hole that is being filled in with concrete. There are two large cement mixers working full time to produce enough concrete to fill the void. It reminded me how I had filled the sink holes and voids in my life with alcohol and that I too needed to secure the stability of my emotional soil. I didn't realise at the time just how much work needed to be done and how big the void was.

Week by week in counselling I started to do the work. It involved putting in the foundations that were missing from my childhood and this was not an instant process. My counsellor gave me the tools, but I have had to learn to build with them. Sometimes I have been building very deliberately and consciously but at other times I have been working without really realising what I am doing. I have had to work out the principles in practice and I now have foundations that are much firmer especially as I am no longer pouring yet more drink into the sink hole.

I noticed that recently the piece of ground which used to have the sink holes is now a beautiful green with a pond so although the ground may never be completely stable it will at least be a place that is appreciated and of value to the community. I hope the same will be true of my life as the unstable ground of my being has been restructured and repurposed.

3.3 Facing up to Shame

I have a better understanding now of the different angles that my counsellor used as she started to work with me. She began by working on my overwhelming sense of shame which was one of the taproots behind my need to drink.

I was ashamed of my drinking and its effects. I didn't want to be a drunk, after all I was a priest, and I had a call from God. I felt ashamed that I just could not live up to my calling as a holy man.

Not only was there shame brought about by my drinking but deep down in my heart was a reservoir of childhood shame. Like a polluted lake that had died and is unable to sustain life. In the mud and the sludge were the shameful things that had been done to me as a child. Gradually through the counselling, the lake was slowly drained as I processed each of these memories. I got them out into the light so that they could dry out and be disposed of. I forgave and received forgiveness. I forgave myself.

I no longer need to drink to forget or to push down the painful memories that drove my shame. I am learning to keep the lake of shame as dry as possible.

3.4 Fear of Fear

Another root of my drinking was fear. What I discovered was that I not only experience fear but I also have a fear of fear. From early childhood, I lived in an atmosphere of fear and as a result, I became fear-averse. I would at all costs avoid the feeling of being afraid and therefore I would try to arrange my life circumstance so that I could circumscribe the fears that come through the ups and downs of everyday life.

The problem is that we can't control our circumstances and without alcohol, I am forced to feel the fear that comes with them. Escape via the bottle is no longer an option so I have to face my fears and the fear of them. It's a double whammy. The feeling of fear and then the fear of those feelings of fear.

In counselling I was able to share my fears, get them out on paper and even identify their source. The way out for me now is not to run away or seek escape when I am afraid. Instead, I now sit with my feelings of fear and my fear of those feelings. My fears are uncomfortable and I don't like them but they don't have to kill me unless I drink.

3.5 Powerful Secrets

As with many people, drinkers or non-drinkers, I had a back catalogue of things that I locked away in the secret vaults of my heart and mind. These buried memories had been squashed down and if I hadn't had the courage and opportunity to share them, they probably would have gone to the grave with me.

Drinking enabled me to keep pushing things deep down inside of myself and it was not until I started to recover that these memories began to surface. This is where my counsellor came to my rescue as she helped me to work through my entire life story and to expose the infection of my emotional wounds to the air.

As we talked through my hitherto secret thoughts and memories, I began to experience freedom and release from the guilt and shame of the past. I had blotted out a great deal of my past and initially, I had very little recall in terms of memories from my childhood. I sort of knew that this was strange and that it indicated something was wrong but I never had the opportunity to do anything about it before.

I went through a season where I would remember things that I had put right out of my mind. These buried memories could surface at any time even in my dreams as the shutters gradually lifted and I could allow the darkness of my past to be exposed to the sunshine of the Spirit. I still to this day get flashbacks and recall from my past as years of suppressed memories gradually surface and get washed up on the shores of my conscious mind.

3.6 Pretty Boys and Gay Men

For the first time in my life, I was able to talk through and process my post traumatic stress that I experienced as a result of attending an English public school.

I had only just turned thirteen when I went to boarding school and was pre-pubescent. I was forced to take communal showers with eighteen-year-old boys, some of whom took a great deal of interest in my physique. I was a pretty young boy with a hairless body and I attracted a lot of attention from some of these older boys who were gay. Initially, I could not understand why they were always in the shower when I was in there, or in the bathroom when I was having a bath.

They were bright and had figured out how to survive and indeed thrive in a school where there was zero tolerance of gay sex. I think that for most of us our life in an all-male boarding school was a very confusing time sexually and there were a lot of casualties.

At times it was really grim and I can still vividly remember one of the boys getting beaten by the housemaster and then removed from the school in a great cloud of shame. He had been caught having sex with another boy. He was a gifted and talented youngman and I think we all keenly felt the injustice of it.

I have met a lot of gay people in the rooms of recovery and I think the struggle that they had in my generation left many of them with some pretty deep wounds that they bathed in alcohol.

3.7 I Am Not

Ordination, particularly in more Catholic circles transmits the idea that when hands are laid on the new priest by the bishop, he undergoes an ontological change and becomes a manifestation of Jesus Christ.

Expectations from congregations and host communities run high and I found myself admitting to my counsellor that I was struggling to meet these high expectations.

I sometimes felt like the magician who was expected to pull the rabbit out of the hat. The problem was that I could not do the required magic tricks and neither could I conjure up a congregation. My performance was continually under scrutiny and I felt that I was being judged against a set of impossible expectations.

Of course, the real Jesus was forgiving and understanding of failure and human weakness, but the Church that bears his name is often another matter. Thankfully this culture is changing but the expectation that the priest will be some form of Jesus is still there.

The irony is that the pressure to be Jesus and my failure to achieve this had driven me further into drinking.

3.8 Heavens Above

When I was training for the priesthood, I saw an old black and white satirical comedy called Heavens Above, starring Peter Sellers as the Reverend John Smallwood. In the film the vicar, a former prison chaplain is accidentally appointed to a very middle-class rural parish which is controlled by a wealthy upper-middle-class family.

Smallwood appoints a black dustman as his churchwarden and sets about passing on the teaching of Jesus that requires putting first the Kingdom of God over against the accumulation of wealth. The vicars love and forgiveness leaves him wide open to abuse and he gets taken for a ride by different groups in the parish who support him as long as they can get what they want out of him.

In the end, they reject him and there is a very telling line in the script at the end of the film where Smallwood says: 'what you want I can't give you and what you need you don't want.' That felt like my story, it wasn't self-pity, it was a prophetic word.

As I sat in the counselling room, talking about this my counsellor helped me to see that given these circumstances, it was not surprising that I had felt the pressure to drink again.

3.9 One by One

What I was enabled to see through this time of reconstruction was that my life had not been the complete waste of time that I had come to believe it to be. The counsellor helped me to move away from my glass half empty type thinking so as to be able to see the positives in my life.

I think alcohol and heavy drinking brings with it a lot of negative thinking. We see through a glass darkly and although I could never see it at the time, alcohol had a depressing and negative effect on my whole outlook on life.

The counsellor helped me to identify some of the good things that I had done particularly in my personal one to one contact with people. Just as I don't know the extent of the damage that I have done in my life, I don't know the true extent of the good that under God I have been able to accomplish.

People with cancer, people with drink problems, people with mental illness, countless bereaved families, loved up wedding couples, delighted new parents, wide-eyed primary school children, miserable school governors, discouraged headteachers and many others who for different reasons God has brought across my path.

I believe that even my time spent in the pub was not wasted as in different ways I was able to engage with people where they were. In terms of community engagement, I was right on it.

I have become aware of what has been good in my life instead of just focussing on the bad. Even my drinking had a good side.

3.10 Renewing the Vision

I could not understand why God had allowed this to happen to me. Why had he allowed me to sink so low? The counsellor floated the idea that maybe this experience would enable me to help others who were struggling with the same sort of things because I had been there. At the time I couldn't take this in because I was still in it, but later this began to make more sense.

What I didn't know all those years ago in my bar room vision was that I would only be able to help those people if I myself was one. God knew that I was one of them even before I did. I wasn't going to be an expert or a consultant, but an insider who knows from bitter experience how difficult it can be to break out of alcoholism once you have come under its influence.

It was to be a little while before it started to become clear that this was my pathway, but now it makes sense, as I have been increasingly involved in helping others caught in the trap of substance misuse. I haven't knowingly helped any vicars with this yet but I guess they are all pretty tight-lipped about their drinking so it's unlikely that I will be besieged with requests for a chat.

My own struggle with alcoholism has given me a heart for the suffering alcoholic and indeed anyone who is on the merry-go-round of the addiction cycle. God seems to bring addicts and alcoholics across my path and if I can't help them myself, I can at least point them in the right direction and enable them to get the help that they need.

Helping other alcoholics in any way I can is now integral to the vision I have for my life. I know that I am not alone in this as many recovering addicts find themselves helping others who are seeking to escape the tyranny of destructive habits.

3.11 Adult Supervision

Over time my counselling changed in its emphasis in the direction of what is called pastoral supervision. Counsellors and psychotherapists work under a strict regime of supervision so that they can debrief and discuss their work and its impact on them.

In my work as a priest, I was fielding some pretty heavy-duty situations in terms of people's problems such as drug addiction, mental health problems, suicide attempts, cancer diagnoses, self-harm, terminal illness and death, including the death of new-born babies and children. I had no professional supervision. I was isolated as a priest and I didn't have colleagues to talk things through with.

For a while alcohol was my supervisor although she didn't do a very good job! The pastoral supervision that I received through the counsellor enabled me to talk through the things that I had just bottled up. I was carrying a lot of guilt, not just about my drinking but false guilt due to unrealistic expectations that I had placed on myself or that had been placed on me by others. It wasn't just my personal issues but also the weight of work-related things that I had not been able to process.

Up until this point I had twenty years of experiences in the priesthood that I had not been able to share with anyone. I was carrying quite a heavy load and this was the first time that I had been able to really download to someone who not only understood but who could also help me to process these experiences. This supervision helped me to start to untangle some of the confusion, guilt and anger that I had been experiencing in some very heavy and difficult situations where I had become involved.

Rather than push it all down with drink I was starting to process my feelings and thoughts in a much more healthy way.

3.12 Fixing People

Somewhere in the course of training for the priesthood, I picked up the erroneous idea that it was my job to fix people. Of course, I only had to look at the rather uncomfortable fact that I couldn't even fix my own drinking problem to see that this was a flawed idea. It was a classic case of trying to take the speck out of somebody else's eye whilst having a log in my own.

We are all broken in different ways and we all need constant repair, but we can't do it on our own. Nobody could fix my alcoholism for me, I had to take responsibility and then in cooperation with God, I had to do the work. I know from my own experience that no one can fix me, but what they can do is put themselves at God's disposal as instruments in his hands to help me.

Like Humpty Dumpty I had taken a great fall, and all the Kings horses and all the Kings men couldn't put Humpty together again. Thankfully I was not alone as God came to my rescue through people and circumstances that enabled me to access the help and the healing that I needed.

I have been fixed and glued back together. There are cracks and signs that I have been broken but I'm still useful to the master, perhaps even more so.

Like a much-valued beaten-up old cooking pot in the hands of an expert chef, I can still be used to serve up some good food at the right time.

3.13 Rebuilding the Walls

My counsellors parting word as I finished my last session has stayed with me and been a constant guiding principle. That word was boundaries. Before coming to counselling I'd not really heard of this word and it was only after much counselling that I started to really understand what it meant.

My upbringing and my drinking had combined to leave me ill-equipped to defend my own boundaries or to know how to keep the right side of other people's. It was only as I met other people in recovery who like myself had weak or non-existent boundaries that I began to see and understand what my counsellor had been driving at.

Drinking erodes and distorts boundaries so that we can end up with the wrong people or put ourselves in the wrong place at the wrong time. I began to see how over the years, right from the earliest days in my family home, drinking had placed me in dangerous positions that exposed me to abuse and harm.

With the benefit of hindsight, I can see that in the past I had been manipulated and used. My childhood and upbringing had blown my boundaries to pieces so that in recovery I wasn't rebuilding broken walls, I was constructing many of them from scratch.

One of the outcomes of this is that I have had to learn to become much more circumspect and cautious in the way I relate to people, as my previous openness and child-like trust had caused me problems.

This has involved the development of much clearer boundaries in all my relationships and this has all been made possible because I am not drinking.

3.14 Slow and Steady

Sobriety is not a quick fix. It has taken a long time and a lot of help for me to sober up and come round from the confusion of drinking. Alcohol was my quick fix particularly in the face of disturbing emotions or difficulties in life. Picking up a drink was so easy and almost instant in its effect but it didn't last. It was only a temporary fix whereas my recovery is slow and steady.

It is taking time to recover and I am learning that in my recovery 'slow and steady wins the race.' Recovery is not a sprint. It is much more like a long-distance event with loads of other people in recovery lining the route to encourage me and cheer me on.

I am still tempted to look for an instant solution to any problem particularly in my emotional life, but I am developing patience and learning to wait. If I wait and I am patient then I believe that the answers will come.

I have to be patient with myself and when I fail, I remind myself that this is a life journey and there will inevitably be times of progress but also times of testing and struggle. My pace is sometimes slow, but I encourage myself with the thought that I am moving forward and not regressing.

Recovery is a life-long project and a constant process of learning and growing. It is sometimes very slow but it is rewarding because even though I fall far short of perfection I can over time see that I am making progress.

3.15 Keep it in the Day

One of the key concepts that have helped me most as I have moved into a life of recovery is the idea of keeping it in the day. I had of course seen this slogan on posters and book covers but it was only at this point in my life that it started to make sense. I have had to learn to keep my recovery in the day and not project into the future.

So much of my life had been dominated by the past or lived in some fear about the future. Slowly I have started to learn the discipline of living in the now. Again, many books have been written about this but the concept and the practice are actually simple. For me, it consists of focussing on what I am doing right here and right now, rather than what I will be doing later, or tomorrow, or next year. This doesn't rule out planning, but it helps to improve the quality of what I am doing in the present which will have the effect of determining a more positive future.

I remember failing to do this one day at the cash machine. I went to draw out cash but my mind was so preoccupied with some future event that I just walked away without taking the notes. By the time I realised it someone else had taken my money. It was an expensive lesson but it showed me the importance of living in the moment and not being fixated on distracting thoughts about the future.

3.16 Hope and a Future

In the first year after hitting my rock bottom not a lot changed outwardly. I was still drinking but at a greatly reduced rate. I don't know how I did it but initially, I was able to come off all alcohol almost entirely for about three months. I knew that it was now very dangerous for me to drink, it was affecting me mentally and I was afraid of what might happen if I continued to drink.

I stayed out of trouble, got on with my work and started to prepare for the future. I remember standing outside the local primary school with the headteacher and she asked me what I planned to do in the future and I said to her 'I want to do a PhD.' Those words surprised me because until I said them as I hadn't really admitted this idea to myself let alone vocalising it.

Only later did I remember how years before I had thought that one day, I would really like to do that. The hidden desire of my heart was exposed. So, I opened a bank account and started to save some money for the first year's fees. I bought some new clothes and developed just a little bit of hope about the future.

This was a struggle because I was still bound by the past, but slowly and steadily through the counselling, the past started to lose its tight grip. I started to get some hope that there might just be a future for me, but I had no idea what that future looked like.

3.17 Rejection

I had to learn to accept life on life's terms and to accept life as it really was not as I wanted to be.

I had to accept that some of the people were never going to like me or accept me and that no matter what I did for them they were never going to be with me or for me. I had to accept rejection and that is hard.

I had spent so much time trying to ingratiate myself with certain types of people but I wasn't one of them and never would be. Their rejection started to become more visible to me and I realised that I had been placating people by desperately trying to please them.

However, no matter how hard I tried or how much of myself I gave I realised that I would never meet with their approval.

My instinctive reaction to rejection from my childhood was to drink but that wasn't working anymore. I wanted to change myself and the situation but I didn't know how to.

I determined that I was going to do something about this and I decided that drinking was not the answer.

3.18 Enough is Enough

One of the last times that I drank too much was at a friend's wake. I went to the wake completely determined that I was not going to have a drink. I was going to have a cup of coffee, a quick chat, and then go home.

When I arrived, I was offered a drink. I said 'no.' They said 'oh go on' and I still said 'no.' Then a beer arrived for me. I took it and began to drink. They all cheered. It was sometime before I left that wake.

What I know now is that I had no defence against the first drink. I knew I didn't want to do this again and I began to see that I would have to seriously think about stopping drinking altogether. It took a few months to do anything about it but I knew I had to stop. I didn't want to get into these situations anymore and I recognised that I was going to need help in keeping away from alcohol if I was going to stop and stay stopped.

I was really sick of waking up sweating and having hangovers, I'd had enough. However, no matter how sick of it all I was and no matter how convinced I was that I'd had enough, by the late afternoon I would be craving a drink, and I often had little or no resistance as evening arrived.

3.19 Life Line

I have to ask myself why it took so long for me to let go of my drinking habit? Why could I not face the fact that it had to go? Why couldn't I have imagined life without drinking? Why could I not have admitted that I had a problem? Deep down I knew that my drinking was unfinished business and yet I couldn't let go of it no matter how much damage it was causing me. I clung to it for dear life as a drowning man holds onto a sinking ship.

The time came for me to let go and reach out for the lifeline. I had to jump ship and take the risk that I could sink. The drink had been my buoyancy aid, my life jacket, and the thing that I clung onto in the storms of life. But now it was taking me down with it and I had to let it go.

When I finally let go, I didn't sink or drown. In fact, instead of sinking, I experienced quite the opposite because as I let go, I started to realise that I could survive and live without alcohol.

I started to learn to cling onto God instead of the bottle. I also discovered that not only was I clinging onto God but that he was holding onto me. He had hold of me on his lifeline.

3.20 Admitting It

It took me until I was fifty-four years old to admit that I was an alcoholic and even then, I had my doubts. I can now laugh about it because the power of my denial was so strong and so delusional, even when it was staring me in the face. I just couldn't see it.

I can now see that certain situations placed me in a position where I just could not avoid getting drunk. Once I got started, I did not have the ability to say 'enough' or 'no' to more drinks. In fact, when the compulsion was on me, I really had no choice.

Until I was willing to admit that I might have a problem and that I needed to seek out help there was little or nothing that anyone could do. Deep down I knew that if I admitted to having a problem with alcohol then I would have to do something about it and I could never again pretend that I wasn't some sort of alcoholic. Admitting it was the beginning of my recovery.

Admitting it became easier once I understood that alcoholism is not a moral weakness but an illness and a 'fatal malady.' Alcoholism is a terminal disease, a silent killer that day-by-day takes the lives of countless numbers of people around the world. It would have taken my life if I had not come out of denial by admitting that I had a problem.

I found that admitting it rather than justifying myself, blaming or making excuses not only worked for alcoholism but also proved to be an effective approach to other issues in my life. I now know how important it is for me to look honestly at situations, asking myself where I am to blame. Where have I gone wrong? Where have I messed up? What was my contribution to this negative situation? If I got it wrong, how could I get it right from now on? I have not only come out of denial about alcohol but also about many other things as well.

3.21 The Decision to Quit

I had vowed to quit drinking so many times but this time I didn't make a vow. Over the previous months, I had become almost allergic to alcohol so that I didn't enjoy having it in my system anymore. I just didn't like the feeling of being intoxicated and instead of relaxing me, it put me on edge.

Somehow, I knew that I had reached the end of the road with alcohol and that it was my time to quit. I planned my exit from the drinking game. I decided to finish the large double magnum bottle of burgundy that my brother had given me and then to stop. So, I had my last drink of alcohol, quite a lot of it.

The next day I had the idea to go to a meeting of Alcoholics Anonymous. The idea just came into my head and I looked it up online. I was worried about my anonymity in my local area so I got on a train and went up to a meeting in the city.

It was in St Michaels church in Cornhill right opposite the Jamaica wine bar where I used to drink when I was a reinsurance broker.

3.22 My First Meeting

I was really excited and scared about attending an Alcoholics Anonymous meeting but I felt very at home when I got there because it was in a rather smart traditional church room and all the people were dressed in their city finery.

It wasn't what I expected at all because the people seemed normal and they all looked so respectable. I couldn't imagine that any of them were real alcoholics and it wasn't all like the meetings I had seen portrayed in the movies.

I was surprised how structured it was and from my background as a priest it seemed like there was a strict liturgy and discipline about the whole meeting. It was tightly ordered and well run but the thing that struck me most was the sharing.

It wasn't people sitting round having a chat and sharing their best ideas with one another. No one was giving advice or trying to tell other people what they should do. The mutual support was given in the form of listening to other people share their experience in recovery from alcoholism.

What really got me was one particular share that was almost a carbon copy of my own life story. He wasn't a priest but his life as a drinker was one that I totally identified with. I knew that they were talking my language and I knew that I needed to come again and find out more.

3.23 Hope

Untreated alcoholism has the power to remove all feelings of hope for the future. The further my alcoholism progressed the more my sense of hope receded. A feeling of continual hopelessness settled on me and followed me like a dark cloud wherever I went.

When I walked out of the door of my first Alcoholics Anonymous meeting, I came away with something that I didn't walk in with, and that was hope. From that point on I had hope that there was an answer to my problem with life as a chronic alcoholic.

I realised that there were many others just like me who had been struggling with the disease of alcoholism just as I had. I walked away from that meeting with conviction that as long as I didn't mess with the program and did what they suggested then I would be alright.

By walking into that meeting, I was admitting that all my efforts to beat this disease on my own had met with defeat and that I was a hopeless case. I could not stop drinking by myself, but meeting these fellow alcoholics who had found recovery gave me hope that I too would receive the gift of sobriety that they had received.

Even on the most difficult of days I now always have hope in my heart because I know that I am being looked after by a loving God who is keeping me safe, giving me hope and a future.

3.24 More Meetings

I was in London quite a lot at the beginning of my research studies so I had the opportunity to attend regular meetings and to learn more from the experiences of others who like me had battled with their desire to drink.

What I didn't expect or know about was the spiritual aspect of these gatherings that were mostly held in the meeting rooms of city churches. I started to realise that I was sensing a presence, a spiritual presence in these rooms. It was the same presence that I knew from my spiritual experiences in church but it was in a room full of alcoholics.

It dawned on me that God was in this and maybe he even liked being there. It must have been refreshing for him, after all those dull and boring church services with the mayor!

It reminded me of the gatherings that Jesus held with the tax collectors and sinners for which he got a lot of flak from the religious folks. I liked the swearing as it gave the whole thing a sense of reality and it was a far cry from the stuffiness and pretence that can surround some of the gatherings that I attend in my life as a priest.

I was really interested in the way that people talked about their 'higher power' as they were explaining the way that this was enabling them to stay sober and to move forward with their lives. I was hooked as I replaced drinking with meetings.

3.25 The Right Path

I wasn't without my doubts about these recovery meetings and I would wonder if I was taking this all too seriously and if I really needed to do this. One day I found myself vacillating about going to a meeting but I decided to go anyway. As I made my way to the meeting, I realised that I was experiencing a sense of God's presence with me. It was as if God was saying 'Chris, keep going, you're on the right path, you are going in the right direction.'

It is interesting that despite all my religious training as a priest and all my experience in the church I really didn't know how to listen to God or to take direction from him. I was self-propelled and took the view that God had given me a brain so I had better use it and make my own decisions. I was religiously informed but spiritually unintelligent because God's guidance could be staring me in the face and I just could not see it.

Practical faith seemed to elude me whilst I was swimming in the deep waters of academic theology and religion. When it came to an everyday working knowledge of God and his will for my life, I was like the college professor who couldn't tie his shoelaces.

3.26 Zero Tolerance

I read somewhere that in the 1930s a member of the Oxford group got some 'guidance' as she was trying to help a chronic alcoholic. The guidance for the alcoholic was 'not one drop.' This proved to be the key to getting that man and many other people sober. When I first encountered this idea, I didn't like it at all. Couldn't I just cut down or moderate? Perhaps I could have a break from drinking for a while and then after a suitable period of abstinence resume drinking at a moderate level?

Deep down I knew that this was just 'whistling in the wind.' I knew it had to be zero tolerance. I had to face reality and that reality was that I had to stop drinking. It was an unimaginable thought but as the evidence mounted, I realised that I was going to have to accept that I could never be a normal drinker.

Drinkers like me never reset or return to factory settings. For us, it's all or nothing and eventually, I chose nothing. Actually, it wasn't nothing as my journey in recovery has been an exciting adventure that I wouldn't have missed for the world.

I still meet the just cutting down idea particularly amongst health professionals who are trying to help those who are not willing to entertain the idea of not one drop. In many other aspects of life, I am very tolerant and liberal but, in this matter, I know from bitter experience that the only long-term solution to alcoholism is to stop drinking entirely.

3.27 The Program

This word is shorthand for the twelve-step recovery program from alcoholism first developed by Dr Bob and Bill W the founders of the fellowship of Alcoholics Anonymous. The steps as outlined in the Big Book of Alcoholics Anonymous describe a method of recovery from addiction that has proved effective in overcoming alcohol addiction across the globe. This program has also proved effective in helping people to recover from other addictive and life-controlling habits such as gambling, drugs, cocaine, overeating, co-dependency, religion and sex.

The program involves 'working the steps' with a sponsor, attending meetings, service in a home group and helping other addicts. This is the program that has helped me to get free from alcoholic drinking and it is this program that sustains my ongoing recovery from the disease of alcoholism.

When I first encountered it, I found it very difficult to get a handle on, because I couldn't understand how it worked. I was used to studying things in theory and then seeing how they worked in practice. This program worked through experience first. The 'big book' in which the program is explained did not make any sense to me when I first read it. In fact, despite being an academic I could not understand it or read it. It took me a long time before I was able to lay aside my prejudice against it and start to study it, not from an academic standpoint but from the position of somebody who was in desperate need of a cure to their alcoholism.

I've continued to kick against the program at various times but I suspect that it's my alcoholism that has been trying to push it out the way as it knows it's met its match. I am of the opinion that there is little chance of good quality long term recovery without a program. I have spent enough time with people in rehab to know that recovery without a program rarely works in the long term.

This program provides me with life-long security because I know that however bad things get there will always be a meeting with people who can help me. As long as I am in the program I am no longer living alone with this disease.

3.28 The Middle of The Bed

Staying in the middle of the bed means that I am less likely to fall out. My alcoholic head often tells me that I don't need recovery meetings and that there are other ways to stay clean and sober. For many years I tried to do it through willpower and serving in the Church, an approach that met with mixed success but ultimate failure.

When I entertain those thoughts of other ways for any length of time, I find myself moving to the outer edges of the bed. I disconnect and cut myself off from the fellowship and the program. For a time, everything seems alright and the experiment goes well but then something happens that triggers my fear and anxiety and then I realise that I can't do this on my own.

As an alcoholic, I need a program and I need to belong to a fellowship that enables me to recover. Without my daily dose of recovery, my disease progresses and I get sick again. I need to stay in the centre of the bed or I fall out and get hurt.

I am not the only one who experiences this as recovery meetings are full of stories of those who have moved to the edges of the recovery process and almost without warning found themselves picking up a drink. It doesn't have to happen but we are all human and therefore we are all fallible.

3.29 St Vedast and St Helen

These two saints' names have played a significant role in my life. At the church of St Helen in Bishopsgate, I came to a living faith and at the church of St Vedast in Foster Lane, I came to experience my faith in such a way that I found freedom from alcoholism. I have a deep love for both of these places and I always enjoy visiting them because of their significance in my life.

St Helen gave me some good theory but St Vedast enabled my faith to find the traction that I needed to gain victory over my addiction. My faith should have been enough to deliver me from my alcoholism and although it helped, I could not find release from my addiction by that means alone.

My God led me to St Vedast and through the help of the group that meets there, I was able to get the information, support and strength that I needed to break free and stay free from alcohol. That freedom that I received initially at St Vedast has gone on to add depth, insight and power to the faith that I had originally received from St Helen.

My lifelong struggle with alcohol has given me a depth of faith and a form of spiritual insight that I would not have been able to access if it had not been in this fight with the bottle. It feels good to win, and for that, I thank God and all the saints, including St Helen and St Vedast.

3.30 Too Dependent

In recovery I realised that not only had I depended on alcohol, I also had the habit of being too dependent on particular people who I looked to for approval and praise.

Throughout my life I had leaned too heavily on certain individuals and had therefore made myself vulnerable to them in terms of exploitation and abuse. Once they realised that I wanted or needed their approval and attention they gained power over me and were able to use this for their own purposes and advantage.

At different stages of my life when drinking I found myself suffering under the influence of people who whilst masquerading as friends were damaging me. I can now see that I was easily led by these people and as a result, I would take a lot of abuse and bullying at their hands.

Alcohol made me vulnerable to abusive relationships and to emotional dependence on people who would use me and exploit me for their own selfish ends.

I still have to be careful about leaning too much on other people and seeking too much of their approval and praise.

The real dependence that I need is dependence on God and that is what I am seeking to experience in my recovery.

3.31 Damaged Conscience

Every time I do something wrong it affects my conscience. For many years I walked all over my conscience but with the recovery of my faith my conscience started to come back. My drinking gave me a bad conscience because I knew deep down that for me it was wrong.

I could argue in its defence along the lines that Jesus drank wine and that Paul said to Timothy to take a little wine for the stomach, but for me it was wrong.

It seems to me that the conscience is a very delicate instrument and if I ignore my conscience there are consequences within myself.

When I continually ignore my inner voice and my sense of what is right or wrong then I experience a negative effect. What happens is that I become hardened in that area of my life. I don't feel as sensitive as I did about it anymore. My conscience becomes seared at the point of my refusal to follow its prompting.

For years in my daily note book, I would write each morning the code TMW. This was my shorthand for too much wine that had been consumed by me the night before. It was good that I wasn't lying to myself but it was even better when I no longer had to write TMW in my notebook.

At last, there was an easy conscience, no more guilt and no more drinking.

April

4.1 Impulse Control

In my drinking, I could be very impulsive and with alcohol inside self-control was often a challenge. I now understand that the part of my brain in charge of impulse control was being put out of action by alcohol so that I would be unable to resist the urge to do or say stupid things.

These were often not bad things just stupid behaviours, but the next day I would often feel ashamed of how I had made such a fool of myself.

Of course, there was sometimes a risky side to these antics and I could act without any real concern or thought about the consequences. I would often feel a pressure or a force pushing me and urging me to say or do something that I later regretted.

In recovery I have been learning more about impulse control and that I don't have to slavishly act on my impulsive thoughts and feelings anymore. I can now pause before I speak or act and I am able to consider the consequences for myself and for others.

This is the fruit of recovery.

4.2 Buried Memories

My conscience is now so much more sensitive than it has ever been. Sometimes memories will surface and I have to face up to the consequences of the hardness of heart that I got into through walking over my conscience in my youth.

Recently I remembered somebody I knew when I was just seventeen. I'd buried their memory and forgotten their name but I began to see and to feel just how much I had hurt them. I saw how I must have damaged that person and hurt their whole family. I must have caused so much pain without even realizing it.

Now all these years later the scales fell from my eyes and my heart thawed as I felt the pain. I found myself grieving for the loss that I inflicted on this beautiful person and the damage that I caused.

My conscience was deeply stirred and I felt truly sorry. I would love to have been able to go and say sorry, but it is so long ago, and I have no idea where they are.

It is no coincidence that I was drinking at the time. I don't blame the drink but I wonder how different it would have been if I'd felt as I do now.

I pray that one day I may have the opportunity to say sorry and to make amends, but for now I make a living amends whenever I offer those close to me, honour, respect, compassion, gentleness, patience, kindness, faithfulness, selflessness and love.

4.3 Saying No

Fitting in was so foundational to my early days of drinking as a teenager. The need to be accepted meant that I found it difficult to say no to things that I should have said no to.

This has continued to be a problem for me ever since as I have often found it almost impossible to say no when I needed to. I seem to be programmed to say yes to anything even if it's obviously against my best interests.

However, since I have started saying no to drinking, I have become aware of other areas in my life where I need to say no.

My habitual inability to say no has caused me a lot of problems particularly when it has meant that I have been pressured or bullied into agreeing to things that I should have said no to.

What I am learning to do is to give myself a bit of breathing space when I am being pressed for an immediate decision. I don't always get it right but I am learning that it is alright to say that 'I'll think about it.' This gives me a bit of time to examine my own motives for saying yes or no. Am I saying yes because it is the right thing to do or because I want to gain this person's approval and be accepted by them? Having given myself a bit of space, I can make a considered decision which could include the word no. I don't even have to give an explanation or an excuse.

My yes can be yes, and my no can be no.

4.4 Any Lengths

It is true that I really do have to be prepared to go to any lengths to maintain my sobriety. My recovery has to come first even when my life gets busy and full which it does. I cannot afford to let myself slide out of the program of recovery that has enabled me to get sober.

It is easy to get complacent with this disease and that's what makes it so dangerous. I have to be prepared to go to any lengths to stay sober and this means that I have to make difficult decisions and choices that can be hard to explain or justify.

I know when I need to get to a recovery meeting or when I need more time in the program and as long as I am true to this sense everything seems to work out. I can get complacent and that is dangerous because that is when my alcoholism awakens and starts to muster its forces. I have to accept that it will never go away.

Alcohol is my Achilles Heel and I will always be vulnerable to its overtures. I cannot afford to change the subject and my recovery has to come first because without it everything else in my life is doomed.

That is why I have to go to any lengths to maintain my sobriety.

4.5 Not Good Enough

My childhood script of 'not good enough' that was constantly reinforced in my school life as a dyslexic, has continued to cause me problems.

Faced with a difficult situation or a problem, I immediately feel that other people are far better equipped to deal with it than me. I defer to them and let others take over, thus denying myself the right to take the lead and to take responsibility for the situation.

My childhood scripting was that I am 'not good enough' and therefore I always thought that the other person would do better than me.

Putting myself down in this way and not stepping up when I should have because of my scripting, has been detrimental to me in my life. It has meant that I have not come forward to do some of the things I should have done and I have allowed less competent people to take the positions that should have been mine. I have then had the frustration of having to watch them do an inferior job.

If I had been operating with a better script, I would have had the confidence to do greater things than I have.

I am now learning that I am enough and that even in the most challenging of situations I will be able to manage and cope well.

4.6 Three Fingers

I like to live on good terms with everyone and I make a conscious effort to view other people in the best possible light. However, I have to accept the reality that there are some nasty people out there who given the opportunity will do me harm.

I don't always know why this is so, but it is true that we will encounter people who not only don't have our best interests at heart but at some incomprehensible level have a desire to destroy us and bring us down.

In the past such people would have exploited my weakness caused by alcohol, but not anymore.

I am learning to listen to my heart and my intuition rather than just operating on the basis of reason alone and I hope that my people radar is better tuned than it was before.

I don't want to be taken for a ride anymore or be taken advantage of by people seeking to exploit my weaknesses for their own advantage.

Of course, the other side of the coin is that I don't want to be a nasty and harmful person myself. The old saying is true when it says that if you point the finger at someone else then three fingers are pointing back at you.

I don't want to harm or hurt anyone by my actions and I seek to keep a firm grip on my motives which can get me way off track. I know that because I am human, I will always fall far short of perfection in my dealings with other people, but I can make progress in the way that I treat other people on a daily basis.

4.7 Accidental Meditation

I accidentally stumbled upon meditation. This happened when I worked in the city and used to pop into a church called St Peter's in Cornhill. It was a Christopher Wren church with very low lighting, and antique dark wood furniture. The wood gave off a wonderful smell and although the church was next to a busy road it was surprisingly quiet. I used to go in most days and just sit there for a few moments in the quiet.

However, these times started to expand as I discovered that once my mind was settled, I could enter a more peaceful state in which I was able just to be and to rest. I believe that God was working in me during these times as I learned to be still and quiet before my creator.

St Peter's became my haven and place of peace as I grappled with the busyness and tension of my life in business at the time.

When St Peter's was closed, I used to walk across London Bridge and just sit or kneel in the side chapel of Southwark Cathedral. Again, the busyness of my mind evaporated and I was able to find deep peace and rest in that place.

I knew nothing about contemplative prayer or meditation except what I learned by experience from just being there and doing it. I think those times of meditation and prayer were highly formative in my call to be a priest even though I didn't realise it at the time.

4.8 Drinking Friends

My drinking friends proved to be more fickle than I would ever have thought. This became apparent when I started to change and wanted to break out of my habitual drinking. I expected them to understand and to encourage me in seeking to broaden my horizons beyond the pub.

However, this was not the case and it became apparent that friendships based purely on drinking are not real friendships at all. In different ways, we were just using each other for our own selfish ends. Some were using the friendship as a way of bolstering their ego, others were using it as a means of entertainment and some were just there to get free drinks.

No one came after me or asked after me when I stopped going to the pub after work. They just carried on without me and it was as if I had never existed. Without exception, I lost all my drinking friends within a very short space of time after I stopped going to the pub. We no longer had anything in common and none of them expressed any interest in the things that I was beginning to explore as I was seeking to escape from the clutches of drink. I think that this is because drinking is basically a selfish activity and many of the people who were drinking with me were just using me as I was using them. I was very sad about this as it wasn't something that I saw coming. I did miss them and I still think about them and their families.

By contrast, the friends that I have made in recovery and in recovery meetings have been amazing. Calling me, helping me, supporting me and being true friends without asking for anything in return.

When I was drinking, I was validating and affirming my friend's drinking habits, but once I stopped, I guess

I was a bit of a threat and my non-drinking raised all sorts of uncomfortable questions about their drinking that they did not want to face up to.

They just carried on drinking and found other so-called friends to join them at the bar.

4.9 Holding On

I'm holding onto God in my heart as I call upon him in the deepest places of my being. I am crying out to him from my innermost self. It's a cry of my heart as I am reaching out to him from deep within. Sometimes I am just offering words or songs of praise. At other times I am asking for help or his presence. I just want to stay connected and not live separately from my creator.

This is the most valuable thing in the world to me. It means more than anything money could buy or anything this world could offer. It is a priceless gift that is so much better than the spirit that I used to hold onto. Gods loving and caring presence in my life is what I hold onto these days.

Holding onto a bottle or a can or a glass is an inferior way of life compared to holding onto the presence of God and the fellowship of his Spirit. I'm deeper with God than I have ever been before and it's what I've always wanted, but I just could not have this and alcohol as well.

It had to be one or the other.

4.10 Falling Short

The gap between what I should be, or could be, or ought to be, is a big one. I fall way short of my chosen ideals and cannot live up to my own standards. I am keenly aware of my failures but not so conversant with my successes. In fact, I tend to dismiss or discount my successes and focus on my failures.

My failure with alcohol has dragged me down over the years and often left me feeling that I could have done so much more with my life. I have to find a balance between glossing over my failures or making too much of them.

We all fail and none of us is successful at everything, including life. Even people who we look up to and regard as successful grapple with their own sense of failure, feeling that somehow, they have fallen short in life.

In any given situation we could nearly always have done more and our best effort will always fall short of perfection. The reality that I have to accept is that I will never live perfectly and that I will fall short of my chosen ideal. I have to live with this, to accept it and to ask God to forgive me and to make good the shortfall.

4.11 Hands Free

Learning to hand my problems over to my higher power and then learning to leave them there has been a major breakthrough for me in my recovery. The first step was handing over the alcohol problem and then leaving it alone. Instead of focussing my attention on my drinking problem I turned my gaze towards the solution in the program of recovery.

I am learning that other problems in my life also find their solution with this approach. Once I have handed over a problem to my higher power, I now try to leave it there. I keep my hands off by refusing to worry and obsess about it. I park the problem and create the space for the God of my understanding to work.

What I want to avoid is taking the problem back by taking my will back. If I find myself slipping back into trying to control the problem I just get down on my knees and hand it back. In this way, I stay hands-free as my higher power relieves me of the problem.

4.12 Intrusive Thoughts

One of the things that I used to enjoy about drinking was the way that alcohol used to shut my thinking down. I have an overactive mind and one of the only ways that I had found to shut my obsessive thinking off was to use alcohol. Alcohol did deliver me some sort of temporary, albeit chemically induced, peace of mind.

Now that I don't use the booze, I have to find other ways to deal with the all too frequent stream of intrusive thoughts that sabotage my peace. These thoughts are like horses galloping across my mind and I have to remember not to get on them because if I do, they take me way off track. I now realise that I don't have to chase down every thought and analyse it.

My mind is a powerful instrument but it can get overheated and if it does then it can start to cause me problems. I find that practical tasks help me to take my mind off my obsessive overthinking and I am finding in recovery that I don't have to chase every thought however intrusive and demanding it is of my attention.

4.13 Trusting and Relying on God

As I face up to every situation in my life, rather than running away and hiding in the bottle, I have been repeating to myself the words, 'I will trust and rely on God.' When I am thinking about the future and my mind starts catastrophising I am challenging these fear-laden thoughts with the idea that 'I will trust and rely on God.'

Seemingly the smallest of life events can trigger my fears. Behind my self-reliance is fear. Fear that I won't get what I want. Fear that if I let go then things will not go the way I want. Fear that God will drop me and abandon me when I need him most.

If I am not relying on God then I am relying on myself or other people and their organisations which often let me down. For many years my self-reliance prevented me from finding recovery because I thought that I must solve my alcohol problem on my own, but I couldn't.

This is my daily conflict between fear and faith. Am I going to continue to let my life be run on fear and anxiety or am I going to learn to really trust and rely on God? Today I will step out in trust and reliance on God in all the situations of my life. Deep down I know that my life works in any circumstances when I can say that ' I will trust and rely on God.'

4.14 Thinking

My drinking and my thinking are closely related. It was only in recovery that I started to be able to unravel my faulty thinking. One day I realised that I had spent the whole afternoon lost in my self-centred thoughts along with their related emotions, and as a result, I had not been present with my family as we went for a walk on a beautiful sunny spring afternoon. My body was there but I was off in my thoughts and those thoughts led me into despair, anxiety, self-pity and fear.

It suddenly dawned on me what people in recovery had been telling me for years. They had told me to ask God to direct my thinking so that it would be free from 'self-pity, dishonest and self-seeking motives.' I realised they were saying that I needed to hand over control of my thinking to God and that as an alcoholic, I would need to submit my thought life to the direction and control of my higher power.

I had always thought that I was autonomous and that I could control everything with my thinking and intelligence, but I realised that left to its own devices my mind could take me way off track, even over a cliff. So now I am praying for God to direct my thinking in every situation of life so that I can be free of self-will and available to be of use to other people especially other alcoholics.

4.15 Next

As an active alcoholic, I was preoccupied with the thought of my next drink and even when I was drinking, I was always lining up the next one. In the pub, I couldn't fully enjoy the drink in my hand because my mind was focused on getting the next round and getting the next drink in.

I was not able to live in the now as I was always living in the next which in my drinking days was often the next drink. I realise that this pattern of not being able to live in the 'now' and living in the next extended into all areas of my life. The next job, the next car, the next home, the next bonus, the next anything as long as there was something more than what I had at the moment.

I've heard it said that alcoholism is a disease of more and that is my experience as I have lived in the 'next' mindset that is always wanting more of my fair share of everything, including, but not limited to, alcohol.

The other day I was at the coast and I just lay down on the sand and looked up at the sky. I could hear the skylarks, the waves crashing on the beach and the seagulls that were flying low from time to time. I watched the clouds and their different layers and the ways they were moving. I was living in the moment and enjoying it.

That is something that I would have found almost impossible to have done before as I was always focused on what was going to happen next.

4.16 Dyslexic Drinking

Once I came out of denial about my alcoholism I started to come out of denial about other things as well. My denial of dyslexia was so strong that it took me three years in recovery as well as a stress-induced stroke to admit that I had a problem.

All my life I had compensated and tried to hide my dyslexia because I was ashamed of it. I felt that it was something that I should be able to totally overcome all by myself. It was a secret and I spent a lot of energy trying to hide it. Slowly I began to accept the fact that I am dyslexic and I was able to receive the help I was being offered in the form of an assessment for a disabled student's allowance.

Halfway through a three-hour assessment with an educational psychologist I found myself completely unable to do some of the tests. As I hit up against this wall it brought back the feelings of embarrassment, shame and frustration that I had experienced at school. These emotions were so painful that I had an urge to just get up and run out of the building.

I now realise that my denial was a self-protection mechanism that I had put in place to avoid experiencing this pain. Once the pain was exposed, I was able to come out of denial and receive the help that I needed.

I am now able to laugh about my dyslexia and I don't have to cover it up anymore. When I hit up against a problem with my reading or writing I just accept the fact that it's because I am dyslexic and that's okay.

4.17 Meditation

Drinking provided me with an altered state of consciousness and in a way, it was a form of spirituality for me. Alcohol was the elixir of life that could take me out of my boredom transporting me into a parallel world and taking me into oblivion.

I was a devotee of the bottle and its spirit had a powerful effect on me as it took me out of myself and into another life. This was not the afterlife but a temporary illusion created by this powerful spirit that took control of me as I surrendered to its deceptive power.

Now that I don't drink, I have to find other ways to get out of my head. I don't mean with substances but with equally powerful means of achieving detachment and serenity. Today I have spiritual practices that take me out of myself and give me the perspective and the peace that I need. I take time out at the beginning of each day to step aside, to reflect, to contemplate and just to be.

It is not always easy to settle, in fact, it is a struggle to break through the barriers of my busy mind, but even on the most distracted of days, there is a reward. The payoff in meditation is often not immediate but comes later in the day when I find myself responding not reacting or being kind when I could have been cruel.

4.18 The Gift of Recovery

I can so easily forget that my recovery from alcoholism is a gift and not a right. It is given by the grace of God and it is given one day at a time. When people ask me how I stopped drinking I have to be honest and say that I don't really know. There was an element of miracle about it and it wasn't something that I had worked for. My only contribution was to take it to such an extreme that I couldn't break free without the intervention of a higher power.

The danger for me is that I can forget that recovery is a gift and I can begin to think that it's all in my power and under my control. The great illusion of control is always waiting in the wings to take over and lead me back out from under the gift of recovery.

The word grace means gift and I know that it is by the grace of God that I have been given the gift of recovery. I do not want to squander this precious gift and I know that the way to keep it is to give it away. The more I give recovery away the more recovery I receive. There is no limit to the grace of God.

4.19 Self-Deception

In an effort to break free from drinking I tried many things including physical exercise. I joined the local running club and ran numerous half-marathons as well as three London Marathons. What people didn't see was that I was using this exercise as a way to blow out my hangovers. I found that a good run could clear the debris of a binge as the oxygen did its work in my system.

I was able to deceive myself and others by pretending that because I was an amateur athlete, I could not possibly be an alcoholic. How could a person who was always out running be an alcoholic drinker?

My running club was a 'Hash House Harriers' club so that too involved drinking. The club motto was 'the running club with a drinking problem' and although this was all very funny it was true. The Tuesday evening training sessions were followed by drinking sessions in the pub that undid all the good work achieved on the run.

In these ways and many others, I deceived myself and let alcohol take more ground in my life.

4.20 Belonging

Even as a small child I was a loner and I have always felt myself to be an outsider. My mother used to constantly remind me how as a small child I was quite content to play on my own and could amuse myself without needing other children or other people around me.

I used to wonder about the word fellowship because although I was a member of a church that used the word, I never felt that I belonged, and often found myself on the margins. I was more of an observer than a participant and I tended to hang back from being able to make a commitment.

It is only recently that I have felt a sense of belonging and that is new for me. It began when joined a local recovery group that meets online and for the first time, I really felt part of the group in a way that I have never done with any other group before.

I am experiencing the fellowship that I had heard about but until now have been unable to access myself. I have found acceptance and unconditional love amongst my fellow alcoholics and this makes me feel that I belong.

4.21 Fruits of Sobriety

One of the most wonderful fruits of recovery has been that I have been able to study and overcome my fear of academic institutions and structures. My journey into recovery coincided with signing up to study for a PhD in theology. In the course of this seven-year sojourn as a part-time university student, I had to face many of my demons particularly my dyslexia and consequent problems with reading for and writing a thesis.

I was able to take a lot of obsessive energy that I had put into drinking and redirect it into the research process. It was a risk that I would not have taken if I had been drinking and there was no guarantee of success even after seven years of study. It was not easy psychologically as I battled with my sense of academic inferiority and there were many highs and lows along the way but I eventually got there.

Achieving my academic potential was a fruit of my sobriety and it could not have happened without the support and encouragement of many people who God brought into my life to help me at just the right time.

One highlight of the journey was when my supervising professor said to me 'Chris you are an academic.' I was just about able to accept this and believe him.

It also would not have happened if I had still been drinking because I would not have had the time or the clarity of mind to invest in the necessary work for a research degree.

4.22 The Plan

The idea that there is a plan for my life was not a new one to me. From my youth, I have had a strong sense of destiny and an awareness that my life is not entirely in my hands.

Strange as it may seem to some people, I believe that my alcoholism was part of the plan of my life just as much as my journey into recovery. Indeed, I would not have discovered recovery if I had not been an addict.

What alcohol brought to the table was confusion and deviation from the plan especially when I sought to run my life my own way by trying to get things to be how I wanted them to be.

My plan was invariably self-centred and my will can be strong as I seek to impose it on a situation. Will power could not stop me drinking, because I couldn't entirely unhook it from my desire to drink. No matter how much willpower I bombard it with it just would not give way because deep down my will was still attached and I was still holding onto it.

What I am doing now is to go with God as I seek his will and his way forward for my life. I am confident that his plan for my life is far better than anything that I could dream up or try to bring to pass by my own cunning or schemes.

I am learning to relax and I am realising that I don't have to make things happen. Of course, things do happen but I don't have to initiate them. Good things happen to me now as long as I don't push and try to impose my will on anybody or anything.

Instead of rushing in to fix a situation, I try to make space for God to move. I look for his way forward and his plan rather than my own best idea. If he initiates and I respond then good things happen.

4.23 Living Clean

Living clean for me is a lot deeper than just putting down the drink. When I was using alcohol, I always had the sense deep down inside myself that I was polluting and poisoning myself. I knew that I was defiling myself but I was powerless to do anything about it.

Now in recovery, I not only stay clean from alcohol but I also experience an increasing sense of inner cleanness as I continue to do the work of recovery. Day by day my God enables me to live a purer and cleaner inner life. My motives, my thoughts, my intentions and my actions are constantly being upgraded rather than degraded.

It feels good to live free and clean from alcohol. Alcoholic drinking was also damaging my body. My teeth, my skin, my hair, and my nails, were all showing the tell-tale signs. But the real damage was hidden from public view as the regular onslaught of alcohol affected my liver, kidneys, pancreas, stomach, throat and brain.

Now that I have stopped this self-destructive life, I am learning to care for myself and to look after myself. Instead of abusing my body, I am appreciating the body that God has given to me. More and more I value my whole self, body, mind and spirit. I now care for it rather than destroying it with alcohol.

4.24 Conceit

In sobriety, I am having to face up to some pretty ugly truths about myself which I would rather keep hidden away from others and even from my own consciousness.

Being conceited means holding an excessively favourable opinion of one's own ability and importance. My alcoholism took me in two directions with this.

Sometimes I would be all puffed up with myself, living in my own imaginary and delusional fantasy world fed by alcohol. At other times I would be the exact opposite and would feel that I was completely useless and a hopeless case. There was little middle ground and I now see that both of these extremes are not the way to live a mentally sane or balanced emotional life.

Conceit is very ugly and I don't even like admitting to having it, but if I recognise it in myself and deal with it quickly, then all is well.

Humility as I understand it involves establishing a balanced view of myself in the light of all available evidence. Not to think too much of myself but also not to wrongly depreciate myself.

4.25 Heading Towards a Drink

There have been times in my recovery when I have been heading towards a drink even when I didn't realise it. This has been when I have backed off and withdrawn from my recovery program. Having made a good start in recovery I have mistakenly thought that I could now do it on my own.

The idea that I am alright now and that I don't need to do that recovery stuff anymore is my warning light that I am heading towards a drink. I cannot pretend that everything is all right and my alcoholism has gone away just because things seem to be running reasonably smoothly.

Recently, I constantly ignored the transmission failure light on my car, I kept driving it until it failed and the whole thing had to be rebuilt at great expense. I need to attend to my alcoholic warning lights as soon as they come on.

The recurring obsessive idea that I am recovered and that I don't need to actively engage with my recovery program anymore is my red warning light. If it comes on, I need to stop, get it fixed, and then get back on my journey in recovery.

4.26 Self-Reliance

About seven years into my journey in recovery I came to the conclusion that I didn't need a program anymore and that I could live a sober life on my own. I lasted about eighteen months and then some life events happened that triggered my fear and I was in trouble.

Then one morning I woke up saying the serenity prayer. I realised just how far I had drifted and at the same time, I knew that this was the cause of my increasing sense of fear. This kicked off a chain of events that led me back into my recovery group.

What happened was that my ego had taken over again and I thought that I could deal with my alcoholism by myself using my own bespoke program. This was just my ego taking back control and running the show once again but this self-reliance did not work as my alcoholism just began to reassert itself in the form of fear and insecurity.

I am continuing to learn that self-reliance does not work when it comes to alcoholism and that without continuous work on a structured program of recovery, I will not be able to prevail against this disease.

4.27 Self-Sufficiency

I think my desperate need to be self-sufficient comes partly from my upbringing in an alcoholic family. I had to look after myself as I couldn't fully trust my significant others due to the presence of alcoholism.

I was grooved in the idea that I could not rely on or trust any higher power other than myself. I could not completely trust my own Father due to the presence of alcohol and the unpredictability and instability that brought into our home.

This self-sufficiency has caused me a lot of trouble especially in recovery as I have found it really difficult to trust and rely on God. Letting go and letting God has been very difficult for me as I have been deeply ingrained with the notion that I must manage things by myself.

Letting go of the idea that I can control my drinking has proved to be a gateway for change in many other areas of my life. Even as a priest, handing things over to God is not something that comes naturally to me, but as

I am seeking to practice the art of letting go and letting God. I am finding that when I do, things go so much better than when I was in charge.

4.28 The Illusion of Control

I spent so many years living under the illusion that I was in control of my drinking, and I honestly believed that I had it under control. The reason that I thought like this was that I was not drinking every day or in great quantities. I could go without alcohol for periods of time and therefore felt that I was not in any way addicted to alcohol. I reasoned that I just liked to drink from time to time and it wasn't a problem.

I really believed that I had it under control and that the excessive drinking days of my youth were over. I went on like this for many years living under the illusion that I didn't have a drinking problem and that it was alright for me to drink even if on occasion I did go overboard.

When I hit midlife, my drinking crept up and, in the end, I was consuming more alcohol than I would have admitted to. The illusion was wearing a bit thin and the consequences of my drinking were becoming more obvious. It was only when I tried to control my drinking and to reign in my consumption that I realised there was a problem.

Day after day I would drink more than I intended to and I couldn't understand why this was so. The illusion of control was starting to break down in the face of the mounting evidence to the contrary. What I didn't realise is that as a teenager I had crossed some invisible line from heavy drinking into alcoholism. I was an alcoholic but I didn't know it and my alcoholism was manifested in my mistaken belief that I could control my alcohol consumption.

It was only when I heard other alcoholics talking about their experience that I realised that I too had fallen for the obsessive illusion that I could control my drinking.

4.29 Moulded by Suffering

Although many people would say it was my own fault and that I did it to myself, I have suffered at the hands of alcohol. The disease of alcoholism doesn't draw much sympathy from those who don't suffer from it because they see it as a self-inflicted illness. For a long time, I agreed with them, and I would relentlessly blame myself for doing this to myself.

What I am beginning to realise is that this disease is like many other afflictions in the way that it shapes the sufferer, so that if, and when, recovery is achieved there is a positive pay-off in terms of what it does to our character. For one thing it is both humbling and humiliating and that fact alone deals some serious blows to our pride and excessive egos.

Alcoholism squeezed vast quantities of self-centred, ego-driven, self-sufficient and wild independence out from me. Through the sufferings of this disease, I have found myself being moulded, shaped, fashioned and formed in a way that would not have been possible for me by any other means. I had to learn the hard way. I had to have my self, bashed out of me by the bottle.

The suffering caused by my alcoholism has proved to be a refining fire burning away much of the dross in my life. Alcohol brought me low and humbled me before my creator. It may have been a pretty ugly road but I now believe that God had a purpose for my soul in all the suffering caused by my alcoholism.

I believe my suffering was fashioning my life so that it could be something beautiful for God.

4.30 Useful Not Useless

One of the consequences of my alcoholism was that I felt so useless. I thought that I had disqualified myself from living a useful life by not being able to get rid of the bottle. I could see other people making a lot more progress in life than me and I felt that my life was on hold. It was almost as if alcohol had pushed the pause button and until I stopped drinking for good, that button was not going to be released.

I could not move any further forward with my life until this issue was addressed. I could no longer bargain with God or try to do a deal by making offerings whilst holding onto the drinking. I could not be of real use in this world until I let go of my drinking and that involved a change that seemed almost too big to contemplate.

I knew that once I picked up a drink, I was useless for anything else. Once I had started, I just had to dedicate the remainder of the day to useless drinking instead of useful work. I felt bad about this because I knew that instead of being useful, I was wasting my time and God's time with this useless activity.

Having quit alcohol, I spend far more of my life in useful and productive ways that are beneficial to myself and others. I feel that my life is now far more useful and that makes me feel better about myself. I am able to gain satisfaction from doing simple things that contribute to my own and other people's well-being.

May

5.1 Putting Something Back

I have found that becoming a volunteer and getting involved in helping other alcoholics in their recovery is a really important part of my own recovery. I am not a professional in the rehab business and I don't have any ambition to become one. What I do have is a lot of first-hand knowledge that I find useful when seeking to help others who are trying to get recovery.

I am not there to preach although I do know a few things from my own experience that could be of some use. I suppose that just by being there I am a sort of visual aid to say that recovery from alcoholism is possible if you really want it. I don't force it on anybody because we are all free to make up our own minds and that is how it should be.

What I find is that my volunteering amongst detoxing alcoholics reminds me of where I have been, and where I could go, if I let up on my program of recovery by believing the lie that after a period of abstinence, I am safe to drink once again. Working with other alcoholics helps me to remember that I can never afford to get complacent and that if I hold onto my own recovery, I can help others too.

In my drinking I was taking a lot out of society but now I feel that I am putting something back. When I help others in recovery, I feel that I am making a positive contribution to society. Every alcoholic who comes into recovery is one less frequent visitor to the hospital, one less petty crime statistic, one less family tragedy and so the list goes on.

This may only be a drop in the ocean but for the recipients of those drops and the ripple effect around their lives its priceless. Every alcoholic who recovers is a miracle and I want to contribute towards that miracle of change.

5.2 Mental Illness

Alcoholism is commonly regarded as a symptom of mental illness rather than being a mental illness in its own right. There is no doubt that many people suffering from various mental conditions use and misuse alcohol as a way of self-medicating and alleviating distressing symptoms, such as severe anxiety. I used alcohol as a way of warding off low mood and symptoms of depression that were increasingly difficult to manage.

Having spent many hundreds of hours listening to alcoholics sharing their experiences of alcoholism, I am increasingly of the opinion that alcoholism should be classified as a mental illness in its own right. My observation is that there are clusters of mental health issues that are more accentuated amongst alcoholics than in the general population. I can't verify this empirically although I believe it would be an interesting and rewarding area for more professional and specialist medical research.

My own experience has been that now I have stopped using alcohol my symptoms of mental illness which included severe anxiety, panic attacks, irrational fear, involuntary shaking, paranoia, low mood, and stress, have greatly reduced. I am convinced that my alcoholism was leading me deeper into a state of mental instability and deteriorating mental health.

Had my alcoholism progressed further, I might well have ended up with a mental health diagnosis as my condition deteriorated. My mental state whilst using alcohol was increasingly unstable and I was at times struggling to hold onto my mental equilibrium and sanity.

I am therefore of the opinion that in my own case alcoholism itself was a form of mental illness for which the main course of treatment was withdrawal, as well as continued and total abstinence from this mind-altering substance.

5.3 Enjoying Not Drinking

I have noticed that people express sadness for me because I can no longer drink alcohol. Someone in my family asked me recently if I couldn't just let my hair down for one evening and have some drinks at a forthcoming family wedding reception. They saw my not drinking as a sad loss and as a negative thing because they felt that I would be missing out.

In contrast to this feeling, I found myself thinking how relieved I was at not having to drink and being able to go to a reception and know that I wasn't going to make a fool of myself and let God, myself and my family down in the process.

This dialogue made me realise how much my thinking about drinking had changed as I no longer viewed it as something that I wanted to do. In fact, I now enjoy not drinking more than I used to enjoy drinking. I get a sense of achievement when I attend a social function and don't drink alcohol. I like being there as a sober person rather than as a drunk person.

One thing I have noticed is that not everyone drinks or wants to drink. I had wrongly assumed that everybody wanted to drink the way I wanted to drink but were holding back because they didn't have what it took to get seriously drunk. I thought they were like me and secretly just wanted to get drunk, but unlike me, they didn't have the bottle to do so. I no longer think like that and I consider my non-drinking life as gain, not loss.

Nowadays I enjoy my sober life too much to want to spoil it by drinking again. I am enjoying life so much more as a non-drinker.

5.4 Wasted Time

I want to make up for wasted time but I have to be careful. My alcoholic enthusiasm can easily set me off at high speed in the wrong direction. Whilst it is true that I have wasted time drinking and recovering from its after-effects, I am now putting time back into helping others to find recovery.

I asked my counsellor the question 'why did I have to become an alcoholic priest?' She said 'well maybe you will be able to use your experience to help others.' At the time I wasn't very impressed with this answer but I have come to see that I have been given a gift of relief from alcohol addiction so that I can help others as they seek to get out of the prison of addiction.

I know what it is like to be trapped in the hell hole of alcohol dependence but I also know that there are some well-travelled escape routes. It takes time to recover and heal from this illness. I have received a lot of help in my journey of recovery and I am now learning to give my time to help others as they too slowly heal from the ravages of this disease. There is no time to be wasted when it comes to the treatment of the alcoholic who wants to get well.

Paradoxically, whilst there is no time to be wasted in helping others, it can feel like you are wasting your time when helping others. The harsh reality of recovery work is that there are a lot of apparent failures as people relapse or give up in their struggle and it can seem like you have wasted all that time on them. It is obviously worth it for those who do make it into recovery and beyond, but I have come to realise that the time, self-sacrificial love and service, given to those who don't make it is equally important.

There is no such thing as wasted time when it comes to recovery.

5.5 Who Am I?

My mother said to me the other day that my father used to say that he never knew what I was thinking. This is true because I never felt safe telling my father what I really thought about anything for fear of his negative judgement.

Through recovery, I realised that this inability to let anyone know what I am thinking has been undergoing some change as I have become able to share myself in meetings. I have been able to be much more honest about what I am thinking and feeling as well as being able to express how I see things.

Before recovery, I was fearful about telling you who I am and this led to a form of dishonesty because instead of telling you what I believed or felt I would just tell you what I thought you wanted to hear. I was so used to operating in this chameleon-like way that I didn't know who I was or what I really believed.

I now see it as a form of dishonesty and I am learning to share what I really think and feel even if I am afraid that you might not like what I say and that as a result, you will not like me.

This fear of rejection meant that I was always putting on a front or an act to keep you from getting near to the real me.

In social situations alcohol provided the fuel to drive this alter ego and effectively prevented me from the honest communication of my true self. This led to further isolation and more drinking.

5.6 Alcohol is a Liar

Alcohol is a liar. It promises so many things that it just can't deliver. Look at any advertisement for booze and you can see that alcohol is making claims that it can never live up to. The sunshine, the beaches, the glistening drinks with happy and beautiful people are a million miles away from the reality of alcoholic drinking.

The advert should have a person sitting on their own in a room with the curtains drawn drinking a bottle of vodka or someone being arrested for drink driving. It should show the university student who is in prison for seven years for a crime that they can't even remember committing because they were in an alcoholic blackout.

Alcohol promises much but delivers less and less because in the end, all it dishes up is pain. In recovery, we stop believing the lies that alcohol tells us and we turn on the liar. The scales start to fall from our eyes as we see the damage that alcohol has done to us and those around us. We see the lies that alcohol has told us and we see it for what it really is.

Alcohol is a liar but in recovery, I am not listening to its voice anymore however attractive the adverts are.

5.7 To be Somebody

My youthful need to be somebody, to be recognised and praised fuelled my alcoholic drinking and inflated my ego so that I needed to become the centre of attention.

Alcohol boosted my alter ego, creating an imaginary self that proved to be a delusion and filling me with all sorts of false perceptions and expectations of myself.

Even when I wasn't drinking alcoholism imbued me with an unrealistic view of myself and my abilities. Alcohol told me how important I was, that I had a right to be somebody and that you should take notice of me.

In recovery, I realised that such alcohol enhanced ego-inflation was delusionary and left me wide open to abuse and manipulation by anyone who would flatter me or stroke my ego. I am learning not to go after recognition or the praise of people. I now take stock when I feel the urge to be a people pleaser or am taken up with the desire to be noticed.

I hold back from jumping into a conversation just to draw attention to myself and I am much more aware of when I am being flattered or manipulated by someone who has latched onto my ego need.

Instead of trying to put myself forward I now seek to be helpful where I can but not to see myself as the answer to everyone's problems. Today I seek to be the person that God made me to be and if that means I live an obscure, unremarkable but obedient life, then that is okay with me.

5.8 No Show

When I was drinking, I could be the life and soul of the party. I wanted you to look at me, to recognise me and to give me your praise. Today, my recovery program encourages me to go in the opposite direction.

It tells me to stay low and not to put on a show. Recovery and the absence of alcohol help me to live a life of humility instead of a life of self-promotion. I now see that my need to be someone and make an impression was rooted in low self-worth. Deep down in my heart, I felt that I was not good enough and I was desperate for external validation, even if it meant doing things just to draw attention to myself.

In recovery, I am building a sense of self-esteem primarily through a life of unrecognised, unsung, and simple acts of service. It involves doing good for its own sake, not to be seen or to gain anyone's approval. I am now happy to let others take centre stage, although not always!

5.9 Drinking Myself Stupid

Without alcohol, I am a reasonable person but when I used to drink, I would often become possessed by the spirit of stupid. Self-restraint, common sense and most forms of balanced or sensible thinking would leave and be replaced by stupidity.

Normally I could make decisions and choices that expressed at least some wisdom and clear thinking, but when alcohol got involved, everything became mixed up. Drinking mixed up my mind and I found life to be increasingly confusing and difficult.

I thought that alcohol was giving me inspiration and original thoughts but these all turned out to be an illusion. In fact, what alcohol did was to stultify my thinking and prevent me from seeing things clearly. My perception of reality became distorted in a way that led me into confusion and depression.

Now that I am no longer taking on board the spirit of stupid, I can live a reasonably balanced and stable life with my thinking no longer clouded by alcohol. I am no longer drinking myself stupid and consequently, I find that I have more self-control and that common sense tends to prevail, most of the time.

5.10 A Love Affair

Like a lot of alcoholics, I had a love affair. I was in love with booze. Alcohol was my mistress and she led me astray. My wife once said to me that when I was drinking it was as if I was having an affair with another woman. I was constantly being wooed and seduced by the bottle, as alcohol would once more lull me into spending more of my time, energy and money on her.

Alcohol got a lot out of me because she knew how to manipulate and control me. I knew the relationship was dangerous and damaging but I just couldn't quite let her go. I could not put her away for any length of time and I would always return for more of what she had to offer.

It was of course an abusive relationship as alcohol began to have her way with me. There was always a price to pay for any time spent in this relationship and it took away much of my ability to love those around me. I had to stop seeing her as she was ruining my life.

Now in recovery, I can put my love where it is meant to be with those I love and those who love me.

5.11 My Tribe

I came out of a recovery meeting at a beautiful old priory in Kent one summers evening. There were a lot of people standing around smoking and chatting in the car park. I remember looking around and thinking, these people are my tribe. We used to hang around in bars but now we are here laughing and joking together in our common journey in recovery.

In my drinking days, I always gravitated towards the drinkers and usually ended up with them. Whatever group I joined, I would by some sort of magic find myself in the company of the heavy drinkers.

I still have an affinity with those who drink and I have sometimes felt cut off from the social side of drinking in the local pub or club. Even if I do go just for a coke, it is not the same, as I am not participating in the ritual and the communion that comes through drinking alcohol with others.

Thankfully I have not had to leave the tribe, I have just joined the non-drinking section who are moving in a different direction in fellowship with a different spirit.

5.12 Hostage to the Future

I am increasingly aware that my level of discontent and restlessness is the result of living too much in the future and failing to keep things in the day. I seem to have been programmed with a future-orientated mindset which means I am always thinking about what is going to happen next or in five-years-time.

The issue for me is how to live with myself comfortably in the present moment rather than being obsessed with what is coming up next. I suppose that what I want is to have everything under control and that includes the future. In the past, I have missed out on so many good things because although I was there in body, my mind was somewhere else.

My family used to say that dads 'not in,' meaning that I was off with my thoughts and not available to them. I feel that I have mortgaged the present for an imaginary future. I have always been looking to do more and achieve more especially in my work. I always want more of what I can't have and can't get, and of course, this has been true with alcohol.

It is said that alcoholism is a disease of more and I would agree with that as it seems to propel me forwards to grasp at what is next instead of appreciating what I have now. Contentment seems to be the holy grail for alcoholics and if I obsessively contemplate and scheme about the future, I find myself more and more discontent.

I am learning to let go of this futile reaching forward and to make the most of every passing moment, but it's hard. I find it easier to live in the imaginary future than with the restlessness and discontent that I often feel in the present moment.

All this tension used to have one simple solution, but now the drinking option has gone, I am having to get on grips with the details of life and not hold the present hostage to the future.

I am learning to take one day at a time and to enjoy one moment at a time rather than wishing my life away in some form of imaginary daydream.

5.13 Real Ale

At one point in my early drinking career, I was a big fan of real ale and I would support pubs that were part of the campaign for real ale. In fact, I would go on pilgrimages to public houses that had allied themselves to this campaign that sought to bring back traditional brewing methods by producing what would now be called craft beers.

I guess this was the closest that I ever got to politics and I felt that by drinking large amounts of real ale in CAMRA pubs then I was doing my bit for the future of the nation.

Some of the beers were very strong and I became an expert at identifying the specific gravity and alcohol content of each of the real ales. Being part of this campaign gave my pub-crawling drink habits a form of legitimacy and almost a sense of respectability.

I was part of a grassroots movement that was seeking to change the nation through changing our brewing industry. In this movement, we became connoisseurs of proper traditionally brewed ales and became an elite group within the drinking classes, or at least that is how it made us feel.

The truth is that for many of us this just provided a smokescreen for our excessive drinking habits and our love for pub life. Whilst there was no doubt many normal drinkers in CAMRA, under the umbrella of the campaign there were many drinkers like me who were in various stages of decline into alcoholic drinking, and I guess that there would be many who have given their lives for this cause, as they have drunk themselves to death.

5.14 Futility, Hopelessness and Despair

My alcoholic condition means that even though I am sober, I continue to wrestle with a gnawing sense of futility, hopelessness and despair.

The inner sense of futility and hopelessness that I can feel, even on a good day, has been a powerful driver for my alcoholism. It is like an inner force that is clambering for release from this world, and many alcoholics end up taking their own lives as they seek to escape this deep inner sense of despair and hopelessness.

Sadly, it is often when alcoholics stop drinking that this sense becomes overwhelming. It's an inside sense that this life that I have lived and will have to live is futile and hopeless.

Like a sea mist, this inner despair can get into every corner of my being so that I cannot see a way through. I believe it is the spirit of despair that comes with my disease and is part of the problem for which I sought an answer in alcohol.

Now that I don't use alcohol, it is revealed more fully, as it is, in all its power, as it exerts its influence throughout my whole being. It is the feeling to which my only response used to be, I must have a drink, but now I have to sit with it. I have to feel its full force, without running away and I see why many people give way to it, as it is the disease at its most raw.

I cannot escape this but I know that the way ahead for me is to stick with it and to move through it. As people in recovery keep reminding me 'this too shall pass,' and I know they are right, even though sometimes it doesn't feel like it.

5.15 Drinking Culture

One of my friends is having his Stag weekend this week and it reminded me just how much drinking is interwoven into our culture. Admittedly the Stag night has developed into the Stag weekend, but it's the same idea, and it is a socially accepted norm. Drinking is what we do to celebrate various rites of passage including times at the other end of life when we hold a wake following a funeral.

As an Anglican priest, I am a chaplain to the culture and that culture involves drinking. For a long time, I was caught up in our drinking culture and my participation in it helped me to do my job. In our culture, social occasions are often drinking occasions and I found a great deal of acceptance as a drinking priest in a drinking culture. My enculturation into my parish was deepened through my drinking and it meant that I was fully engaged with the culture and very much part of the furniture.

In many ways, I think that over the years God used my drinking for the good as I was involved in the various local rituals and rites that involve drinking alcohol. A lot of people like a vicar who likes a drink as this provides some common ground and a sense that you are a normal human being. There is a sense in which by drinking I was speaking the language of the people God sent me to.

One of the sad things about having to stop drinking was this loss of connection with the culture and the people whose company and friendship I had enjoyed. I still like to pop into the local bar from time to time but it's not the same now that I no longer drink. I feel a sense of separation and distance in a way that I didn't when I was drinking alcohol.

5.16 Compromised Faith

I thought that by becoming a priest there would be less pressure to compromise my faith. I wanted to live a life that was true to my faith and I thought that by entering the church as a priest, I would be able to avoid the compromises that I was faced with in my life in business. To my great surprise the temptation to compromise my faith was still there when I became a priest, but often in a different form. The temptations to bend the truth or give a false impression were still there, as was the temptation to get drunk.

I remember going to a dinner party as a new priest and getting stuck into the olives, the champagne, the wine and the schnapps, only to find myself hanging over the toilet bowl all night and then having to get up to lead and preach in church on Sunday. Alcohol took me into situations of compromise where my ideals were put on ice so that I could drink and behave in whatever way the alcohol directed.

I didn't want my will to be split and divided in this way, but it happened, and I had to live with the guilt and shame of falling short of the standards that were required of a man of God.

What I have realised is that the Church that I joined is itself a compromised one, because at the end of the day it has to go along with the cultural norms of society, rather than being able to stick with its core principles.

It is therefore not surprising that I have found myself in numerous situations where my faith has been compromised.

5.17 Letting Go

Letting go of my drinking has opened the door for letting go of other ideas that have held me back in life. I have had to learn to start living in a different way from how I used to live before. One particular set of circumstances in my life showed me the importance of letting go of my way and relying on God's way.

I was summoned to the university where I was studying for my PhD and told that the department, I was studying in was being closed down and the academic staff were being forced to move on. I was halfway through my time and I was initially angry but a strange thing happened to me. I started to realise that the whole situation was a test of my sobriety and that I needed to learn a new way of operating through this crisis.

I decided to accept the decision rather than resist it or fight it and as I did so a series of miraculous events took place. I was able to upgrade to PhD status, I was transferred to a really prestigious faculty, I was given two amazingly gifted and caring supervisors and I was awarded a disabled students allowance, which resulted in my getting a new desktop computer and a proof-reader for my thesis.

This all happened because I was willing to let go and to trust God for the outcome. Two years later I was awarded a doctorate for my thesis and I don't think that would have happened if I had held onto my own idea of what I should do.

5.18 Adult Children

I grew up in a militaristic household as my father had been moulded and shaped by the military. We would be woken up very early on weekends as my father embarked on his Saturday morning routine of chores which included polishing all our shoes so that they would pass any army inspection parade. I would go round to friends' houses and find that none of them were out of bed when it seemed to me that it was already the middle of the day.

There was also a dark side to the military regime particularly in the realms of harsh and unjust punishment. I remember when I was about four years old and my baby brother fell over and cut his head on a pile of bricks in the back garden. My mother was out and my father was looking after us. He heard my brother scream, saw the deep and bloody cut and then he hit me hard around the head so that I too fell back screaming in pain and from the injustice of it.

My dad was himself an adult child of an alcoholic family and the disease was not slow to manifest itself in my upbringing as a good clout was the solution for the slightest of errors even when I wasn't to blame.

I was very well drilled and I was extremely obedient as a child but I was being physically and emotionally abused by my father who was just passing on what he had learned about parenting in his family.

Alcoholism and abuse often seem to go together and they seem to be passed down the generations like ginger hair or freckles.

5.19 Vows to Quit

Over the years I made hundreds of sincere vows to quit drinking but I always went back to it, so that in the end I gave up giving up. This pattern of an earnest desire to quit followed by complete caving into my intense ongoing desire to drink made me feel like I would always be destined to fail. Repeated attempts to stop drinking followed by relapse became an almost constant feature of my life.

This pattern of relapse followed by reform and then relapse again made it difficult for me to believe that I would ever be enabled to quit drinking. I found it difficult to believe myself as I really meant it at the time when I said I was going to quit. In that moment of the vow to quit, I would mean it but that commitment would get eroded so quickly.

I fully identify with people caught in the cycle of serial relapses and the belief that it is never ever going to be different. Eventually, I started to think that I was one of the unlucky ones who would never be able to break free, but something happened to me that brought about the change that I needed to make in my approach.

The change for me came when I followed up my vow to quit by seeking outside help. I decided to get help from people who knew what they were talking about. That is other people who had the same problem. It was that simple act of reaching outside myself for help that enabled me to find the release that I had been looking for.

As long as I was just trying to do it on my own and to fix myself it never worked. My vows to quit had always been followed up by action and that action was to drink. When I followed up my vow to quit with the action of joining a mutual support group, I found the ongoing freedom that I had been trying to find on my own for years. As I have thought about it, I realise that by reaching out to others, I was in some strange way reaching out to God as well.

It was prayer in the form of a vow followed by the right action.

5.20 Contemplative Prayer

As a priest in the Church of England, I am expected to pray every day as part of my job. Over the years I have tried many ways and methods as I have sought to make prayer central to my life.

At the moment my practice is to spend the first part of every morning in prayer and meditation, as I seek to embrace a life that is in tune with the heartbeat of God. Getting to this point has been quite a journey as I have lived through more than a few seasons when I have found it difficult to pray at all. I guess that is all part of the learning process when it comes to praying and connecting with God.

These days I don't say very much to God and focus more on what he might be saying to me. I suppose you could call it listening prayer or contemplative prayer, but the process is the same. It involves being still, which can be quite difficult first thing in the morning when your mind is racing through all the things that have got to be done.

Contemplative Prayer for me is not about emptying the mind, rather it is about engaging in the process of seeking to still my mind before God. It's never quite the same each day as sometimes it seems easy but on other days, I find it almost impossible.

Some days I awake praising God, conscious of his presence and just repeating his name over and over again. But on a normal day, it involves more work, in self-examination, confession, spiritual reading, and waiting on Him in stillness and silence. I usually conclude my prayers with a few set prayers that I have committed to memory because they remind me to seek and to do the will of God in all the affairs of the day.

I don't believe in formulas when it comes to prayer as for me it is a relational practice because God is my friend as well as my boss. My day is always lacking and often falls well below par if I am prevented from spending the beginning of the day with God.

5.21 Alcoholism Arrested

My alcoholism is arrested but I am not cured. I now know that no matter how long it is since my last drink, I can never safely drink alcohol again. This is the missing piece in many people's recovery programs and it was the missing piece in mine. Logic would say that after a long period of sobriety, a careful return to moderate and limited drinking would be fine. This logic sounds good and appealing but in practice, it just doesn't work.

Alcoholism is not logical in fact it defies all logic and common sense. Even after years of sobriety and abstinence, I know that I cannot take a drink because it would just kick off my disease again. Alcoholism is a disease for which there is no known cure. What has happened to me is that my disease has been arrested as long as I don't set it off again by drinking alcohol. It's that simple but also that difficult because my alcoholic mind constantly argues with this idea and wants to rebel against it.

The disease of alcoholism inside me is like the fifth column. It is the enemy within that wants to destroy me from the inside out. I've heard people say that alcohol wants them dead and I know what they mean. It's a nasty and aggressive disease that is just waiting for the opportunity to take over again. It's like shingles, it waits until the body is weak and vulnerable and then springs into action. No real alcoholic can afford to ignore the fact that alcohol is not to be ingested. If it is the results are always disastrous.

A heavy drinker can get away with it but not an alcoholic. I don't want to take any risks with this neither do I want to engage in further research by drinking. I wish I could be cured of my alcoholism but I can't, it's incurable. However, I am glad that this disease is arrested and that I don't have to let it destroy my life any more than it has done.

5.22 Public Image

The difference between the outer self and the inward reality can be very costly. I've heard it said that alcoholics tend to present their stage character when drinking. This is not the real self but a protective shield to keep people out so that they won't get near the real person behind the mask. People are not stupid and they know when they have not met the real you and that they have not connected with your true self. Keeping up appearances, and projecting an image or reputation in this way is hard work.

I am glad to say that the disconnect between my public life and my personal private one is much more united these days, and it feels so much better. Being honest is much easier than trying to project some sort of front, and far less damaging to those around us.

One of my friends told me about his alcoholic dad who was a big shot and an influential player in the art world. But when he was at home, he was a complete mess and wreaked havoc on the emotional life of his boys, who both became chronic alcoholics themselves. His drinking meant that whilst he kept up a good façade at work, he was unable to meet the emotional needs of his children and wife having directed all his energy into his work. It is this performance mentality that drives a lot of functioning alcoholics who use alcohol to help them to keep up appearances through their work. The show must go on and if it takes loads of drinking to do it, then needs must.

Performance orientation is a feature of many alcoholics who are able to keep their working life together but not much else. Wives, children and families all have their lives sacrificed on the altar of alcohol-fuelled working habits. When I stopped drinking, I realised just how much I had fallen into this trap, even as a priest. The church is a greedy monster and will gobble up everything you've got to give, and more. Workaholism and alcoholism go together, even for priests.

For the still suffering but functioning alcoholic, appearances and public image have to be maintained at all costs even though behind the scenes the back of the house is falling to pieces.

5.23 Acceptance and Change

It is the power of acceptance that brings radical change. When I finally accepted my alcoholism and that I truly was 'one of them', then the doorway to change opened immediately. Although I didn't understand it at the time it was as if I was transferred into a different mode of existence. Something happened to me when I accepted that even though I wasn't sitting on a park bench with a can of super strength lager, I was actually an alcoholic. Accepting this reality placed me in a position to change and that change started immediately. It was a battle of the wills. My will against Gods will and eventually I gave in and he won. I'm glad he did because my way was only heading for disaster and misery.

I still hit up against situations where I am being asked to change and I don't like it. I want to stay as I am and I want things to be the same because it makes me feel more secure. I resist and fight to keep things the way that I want them and I get angry that I am being asked to accept a different course of action or a different way of thinking about a situation.

Acceptance doesn't come easy for me and I often find myself fighting and resisting change until I realise what I am doing. Once I get over the hump and work through acceptance into change then things usually work out much better for me. I look back and think to myself why did I hold out against that for so long? The answer is that it's because I'm an alcoholic. Lack of acceptance comes as a bundle with the alcoholic condition and I have to accept that.

I can even laugh about it now when I think back to how stubborn and stupid, I have been about refusing to change so many things, including but not limited to my use of alcohol.

5.24 Spiritual Bank Account

Self-reflection, meditation and spiritual reading are all part of my investment in the spiritual aspect of life. Each day I try to make a small deposit in my spiritual bank account which doesn't seem much at the time but it is cumulative and when my spiritual bank account is in credit, I know I have the resources to meet the most challenging of days.

In fact, it is only when I'm out in life that this investment in the spiritual realm really pays off because

I find that I have a different perspective that is not a purely material one. Even in the difficult and testing things, I am able to see that there are lessons for me to learn and I can accept them as a challenge and an opportunity to grow spiritually.

I am learning the discipline of standing back from a situation and looking for the thing that God might be trying to work in me through it. It is easy to conclude that not much is happening spiritually especially when there is no immediate or obvious change, but it is like investing in a savings account that accumulates a deposit that is there even though you are unaware of it most of the time.

I am slow to tie up my prayer with the answers that come from those prayers and I think this is often because there is often a time delay or the prayer is answered in a way that does not, at first sight, seem to relate to the original prayer. I also forget what I have prayed for and therefore I can miss the fact that the prayer has been answered.

Sometimes the answer may come in a way that I am not initially happy with and it may not be the way that I scripted it in my mind when I prayed. The answer is sometimes a clear no from God and that can be difficult to accept at the time but very often as I look back, I can see that by blocking the way God has prevented me from doing or saying something that would have been damaging to myself or others.

All I have to do is to make a small deposit each day and I find that I have the spiritual resources when I need them.

5.25 Proud Dad

There's a tiny photo of me with my dad outside our house in Wales in 1963. My dad was immaculately dressed and I too was suited, booted and very smart. In the picture I have a big grin on my face, my dad is holding my hand, and he is looking very proud of his son. It all looks brilliant and so it was, but something happened.

As I got older my dad's pride in his son took on a new direction as he wanted me to be better and superior to the children of his friends. My dad was very intelligent and had a huge amount of unrealised potential so he started to express his own ambition through me and my younger brother. Almost overnight he took an interest in my schooling, took me out of the state education system and sent me to private school.

I had to be tutored to get into preparatory school and whilst I was reasonably intelligent, I was also dyslexic, a condition which would prove to be the fly in the ointment throughout my educational life.

My dad worked really hard to earn the money to pay the fees but the problem came at the beginning of each school holiday when the bill and the reports would arrive. I remember living in fear and dread of the report's arrival through the post and I would go and hide up the road until my dad's rage had subsided as he read page after page of comments like 'must try harder.'

In order to try to improve my performance he completely withdrew all forms of praise and approval. From then on, I would strive and work for his approval and try to please him with my performance, but to no avail. I was not and could never be good enough. What I needed was acceptance, affirmation, approval and encouragement but what I got was scowls, temper and crushing criticism.

From the best of intentions, he smashed my self-esteem to pieces and I still struggle when I am in situations where I am being criticised or run down for my performance. Low self-worth was a driver for my drinking and it's been quite a battle in recovery to undo some of the damage that was done all those years ago by my well-meaning proud dad.

5.26 Self-Pity

I gave myself a bad day yesterday because I started to feel sorry for myself. I looked at my circumstances and went down a path of thinking that led me into self-pity. It made me feel so bad and so low. It is only today that I can see how this happened.

I allowed myself to follow a negative trail of thinking about my life and about myself which took me to an emotional state in which I experienced fear, insecurity, discontent and disease. I did have the self-consciousness to pray for help and thankfully the obsessive thinking and the feelings did eventually pass, but it was uncomfortable.

I need to guard my thinking against self-pity and challenge it when it rises up within me. There is no need to walk around feeling sorry for myself and it only makes me feel bad. If I can take the focus off myself and seek to help others then I know that all will be well.

I need to remember to take the antidote which is gratitude. There is nothing that dissolves self-pity faster than sitting down and writing out a list of things that I am grateful and thankful for. A friend of mine taught me how to do this as it was something that he had learned in his recovery. I guess it is one of the most powerful tools in recovery and a lot of different recovery groups use it.

The friend who taught me just sat down with me and read out his gratitude list. He didn't actually have many things or people in his life so I was greatly humbled as he set off thanking God for his phone and his lunch. I had a lot more in my life but I just couldn't see it with my negative glasses on.

If I remember to do it, I can eject self-pity with just twenty things on my gratitude list.

5.27 Manipulation

The alcoholic life made me vulnerable to people who would use my weakness to manipulate and control me for their own purposes. Manipulation involves trying to control or influence people to get your own way without them realising it. It often involves using devious or dishonest tactics to control a relationship or a situation.

My alcoholism made me an easy target for those who wanted to manipulate me to get what they wanted or needed from me.

Only now in recovery am I beginning to detect when I am being manipulated or used by someone. I am no longer so easily coned into agreeing to things that go against my best interests and I have been learning to say no to people who are trying to get me to do and say things that I really don't want to do or say.

I still find myself under pressure from people who want to manipulate me and it can still be difficult to detect or to resist their manipulative ways. However, without alcohol in the picture, I now have a much better chance of detecting manipulation and dealing with it sooner, rather than later, when the damage has already been done.

Now when I find myself tempted to saying yes to somebody too quickly, I pause and ask myself why I am feeling such a strong obligation to fulfil their request? My latent desire to please is so strong that I can find myself saying yes to things before I have had a chance to weigh up the situation properly.

I have had to teach myself to say that I just need a little time to think about it. If people don't want to give me that space, I now know that I am probably being put under pressure and I need to be careful.

5.28 What I Need

It is said that alcoholism is a disease of more. We always want more and enough is not enough. We can get envious of those who have what we think we want. In recovery, we start to see things differently and we begin to appreciate what we do have rather than always grasping for more.

It is true that I don't have everything I want but I do have what I need and I am finding that I want less and less. I am learning to be content with what I have and where I am in life. I appreciate the gifts and abilities that I have been given as well as all the good things that have come my way.

I am not a victim and I refuse to engage in self-pity. I have much to be thankful for and a lot to celebrate. I no longer dwell on lack or compare my lot in life with others. I have what I need and I am no longer craving or striving for more.

With this attitude, I find that the things I need in life come my way naturally. Things come to me as I need them rather than me having to go after them and grab them or snatch them from somebody else.

My sense of alcoholic discontent has lifted and I am learning to be grateful and pleased with my lot in life. I appreciate and value my life now instead of tearing it down and destroying it with alcohol.

I am finding that God goes before me and knows what I need even before I have become aware of it. I am richly provided for and enjoy many blessings that even money can't buy.

I am where I belong, I have what I need, and I appreciate what I have. I no longer think of myself as a victim of circumstances but I see myself as someone who lives in blessing and favour. I know what it means to count my blessings, only there are too many to count.

5.29 Feeling the Presence

I know that it is difficult for people who don't feel God's presence to get this but I really do feel God's presence. I have to qualify this by saying that I don't feel it all the time and the feeling comes and goes. For the last five days, I have been feeling that God is keeping himself at a bit of a distance and I have felt quite separated from his presence but this afternoon whilst I was walking, I suddenly felt it. It was momentary but so good and reassuring to know that God is still with me.

I know that when I was drinking the sense of God's presence would diminish as the alcohol blocked my sensitivity to the presence. Nowadays I crave the felt presence of God like I used to crave the presence of alcohol. I no longer thirst for a drink instead I thirst for God's presence.

I know God is always there like the sun but it gets cloudy, overcast and at times dark. It is then that I live by faith. I trust that even though I can't see him or feel him he is still there. Then just when I am not expecting it the sun breaks through the clouds and I am suddenly aware of the presence of God with me. It can happen anytime and anywhere.

I often experience His presence when I am in recovery meetings with other addicts and alcoholics. Quite often I feel him when I am on the way to a meeting. I think of it as the fellowship of the spirit and the fellowship of suffering.

I am convinced that God is not confined to buildings or religious ceremonies. He is a free spirit and moves just where and when he wants. He is untamed and cannot be domesticated. He comes and goes just as he wishes and this makes for an interesting life.

5.30 True Identity

We tend to identify ourselves by external things like our job, achievements, abilities, disabilities, class, gender, looks, size, cars, houses, money and even tattoos. But whilst we use those things to define us, they are not who we are. We are directed to look at the outward appearance of people, but God looks at the inside of us, the heart. He sees what's really going and he knows us better than we know ourselves.

Our suffering is often unobserved or unnoticed even by those who are close to us, but God sees every sadness, every wound and all our tears. We hide to protect ourselves and put up a front to keep others from seeing our pain. Our true identity is therefore masked but the image that we put up is still being penetrated by the gaze of our higher power. Nothing is hidden from the eyes of God, he sees it all, all of us, the good, the bad and the ugly. Whilst we look at the outward appearance God looks at the heart.

Meditation for me involves getting into alignment with him by seeing what he sees and agreeing with him. This is true peace as I find myself much less internally conflicted. My outside and my inside become more lined up and instead of being out of sync, I find myself moving in step with the Spirit of God.

As I become more aware of who I really am on the inside and of my God-given identity, I am learning to live from my true identity as a child of God and not from the identity that society brands me with.

Finding out who I really am in this way, and then learning how to live out of that identity, is one of the most liberating experiences in my recovery.

5.31 Doing Nothing

I've got a postcard on my wall with a picture of a hamster on it. The card says, 'it may look like I'm doing nothing but in my head I'm quite busy.' This seems to me to sum up the alcoholic mind. Stilling my busy mind and getting it to shut up has been a big challenge for me in the process of recovery.

The idea that I could sit still was not alien to me and when I had achieved this at various times in my life, I knew how wonderful it could be. Don't get me wrong it wasn't always Nirvana, but there was something going on even in the most snatched moments of peace.

As a teenager, I remember waiting to file out of school chapel and sensing a peace that I wanted to hold onto. I didn't want to leave it as it was so precious but although I liked it when it happened, it never occurred to me to develop it further. It has always been much easier when

I have fallen into it by accident or stumbled across it casually.

Stillness is so difficult for me. I know deep down that this is the very thing that I need but I just can't turn my thinker off. Recently I have been experimenting with being quiet for five minutes at a time. I got into this through a recovery group that I belonged to where the session would always begin with five minutes of silent meditation. For a group of recovering addicts, this was a significant feat but it worked and it got me into the habit.

I remember in the group meditations I used to be quite distracted but slowly I started getting into it and found myself really looking forward to it. Doing this with the group gave me the idea that I could do it on my own at home. So, what I do now is to pause for five minutes, set the timer on my phone and begin by meditating on the words 'be still and know that I am God.'

At a recent wedding reception, it was all getting a bit much especially as I was surrounded by heavy drinkers. So, I snuck off back to the car for a couple of sessions of five minutes of silent meditation. It really worked and I felt my spiritual batteries got recharged so that I could navigate the rest of the proceedings without the thought of a drink.

With meditation, once I get into it, I often want more, and when I leave a session, I regularly come away with much more of Gods peace, stillness and presence than I started with.

June

6.1 The Illusion of Control

I have a postcard by my door which says 'nothing is under control.' It took many years to accept the fact that I could not control my drinking. The more I tried to control it the worse it got. Weeks of enforced abstinence would be followed by periods of even more wild drinking than before. It was a truly baffling situation until I came to accept that my drinking was out of control. I had to come to terms with the fact that for reasons I didn't understand I could not control my drinking.

Of course, I now realise that there are so many other situations where I am not in control. The postcard by my door is a constant reminder to me about the illusion of control.

I remember years ago the finance director of the company I worked for came back from a six-week intensive management training course. He sat down at his desk and said 'now I am in control.' The course had so boosted his confidence that he felt that he could now control everything. I remember thinking at the time that he might be heading for disappointment. Needless to say, his illusion of control soon evaporated in the reality of the business world.

As I have let go of trying to control my drinking, I have found that the same approach works in many other areas of life where I had assumed that I was in control. This doesn't mean that I abdicate all responsibility it just means that I move in life with the awareness that I may well not be able to control the outcome of the situation in front of me. This approach saves me a lot of wasted emotional energy and fatigue.

I no longer give so much attention to fretting over situations that are not going my way. Instead, I accept them as they are and then look for appropriate solutions in the light of the reality in front of me.

I am not sure I want to go as far as saying that 'nothing is under control' but the reality in my life is that I am in control of far less than I used to think I was, and that is acceptable to me.

6.2 Drifting Away

As we get our lives back after active addiction, it's easy to take the foot off the gas in terms of the ongoing work of recovery. Life starts to take off and it's easy to forget that everything we have is built on the foundation of meetings and the basic principles of recovery. Without regular involvement in recovery work, it's easy to drift away.

All of us in recovery hit times when life just seems too busy and too full to be bothered with meetings and the ongoing maintenance of our program of recovery. As long as we are attentive to the program, we are like a barge tied up to the docks on a fast-flowing river. But as we let go of the program, we get our mooring severed and we start to drift downstream. Before we know it, we are miles away from the security of our mooring. We are in danger of getting wrecked as the tide takes us towards the estuary and the rocks. We can move so far away without even realising it. Silently we drift and we wonder why it is so hard to get back.

Many never come back as they succumb to the inevitable temptation to take the fatal experiment of the first drink. How did I get here? How has it come to this when my life was so on course? The answer is that we drifted away and got swept far out to sea without even realising what was happening until it was too late.

6.3 Looking after Myself

Alcoholic drinking takes its toll on the body. It's a destructive form of self-harm that often leads to premature death and suicide. We delay or avoid eating food so that we can get a bigger hit from the drink. We live on painkillers and stomach pills. Many alcoholics chain-smoke and use other substances. Day after day our bodies take a massive and punishing beating as we pour yet more booze down our throats.

But in recovery, we stop abusing ourselves. Slowly we begin to look after ourselves instead of beating ourselves up. We begin to take an interest in our health. As we find ourselves, we can look in the mirror and we are no longer ashamed. However, even in recovery, I find that I need to be careful and to keep looking after myself.

I spend a lot of my life looking after other people and I tend to put their care and their interests before my own. This is all very admirable but what I have realised is that in doing this I can easily neglect myself and my own legitimate needs. Instead of immediately overruling or dismissing my own inner voice, I am learning to ask the question, what's right for me in this situation?

In the past, I have paid a heavy price for ignoring myself and my own sense of what I need and want. I now know that my needs are important and whilst they are all open to negotiation they need to be listened to. I have realised that this habit is a form of self-neglect as it can cause me to fail to look after myself as I put others interests ahead of mine.

6.4 Sunshine Drinking

In the late 1960s, my Father and Mother took me on holiday to St Tropez in the south of France. It was quite a culture shock and an introduction to a sort of life with far fewer boundaries, which of course included drinking.

My father took us on a cultural outing to the local wine cooperative where he bought many litres of draught rose which was really nice to drink. There were also trips out for Grand Marnier Crepes and French beers served in the cafes and bars on the seafront where the people on the luxury yachts showed off their wealth.

Drinking in that environment with the sunshine and sense of freedom made a big impression on me. I was encouraged to drink alcohol because my parents felt that it would demystify it and enable me to learn to drink sensibly.

It was so different from drinking in Britain which seemed like an industrial process compared to the relaxed atmosphere of the French cafes. It was all very glamorous and from that time onwards I always enjoyed sitting in the sun drinking outside bars and pubs.

These days it still turns my head when I drive past a pub in the summer sunshine and see people sitting outside drinking glasses of cold lager.

6.5 Feel the Feelings

My toxic home life left me feeling extremely uncomfortable in my own skin. Often nervy, on edge, and generally ill at ease for no particular reason. I remember these feelings creeping up on me in my mid-twenties especially at work. I went through a phase of feeling very anxious and the high-pressured business environment seemed to trigger my feelings of dis-ease.

The arrival of these feelings came with a sense that I would never feel any different. At such times, I would habitually reach for a drink because I knew it would change the way I felt. I knew that if I just had a couple of drinks, it would take the edge off my anxiety and sense of fear.

It has taken me a long time to learn that rather than reaching for a drink, I just need to remind myself that this too shall pass. Feelings are like the weather; they will eventually change even though it doesn't seem like it when you look out the window. As long as I sit it out, and as long as I don't pick up a drink to change the way I feel, I will survive.

Looking back, I probably put too much emphasis on how I was feeling and this was a snare. Feelings come and go and I have spent too much time using alcohol to avoid feeling things. I now accept my feelings no matter what state of dis-ease they may leave me in.

Importantly I no longer allow my feelings of fear to hold me back from taking legitimate risks and doing what I know to be the right thing even though I am feeling the fear. I now allow myself to feel the fear and do it anyway.

6.6 Impending Doom

Growing up in an alcoholic home left me with a strong sense of impending doom. The insecurity of my home deposited within me a constant feeling that something was just about to go wrong. It was difficult to enjoy good times because I was always haunted by the thought that things were too good and something bad was about to happen. I always had to be on guard and ready for the next crisis which meant that I found it difficult to relax and I was stressed out a lot.

Even when things were going well, I was often plagued by a sense that this was too good to be true and something must be about to spoil it. Just as my father's mood could turn on a sixpence from sunny and upbeat to morose and angry, so my sense of wellbeing was always destabilised by intrusive thoughts of the possibility that things might turn bad at any moment.

Alcohol provided temporary relief from this feeling of insecurity and the fear of what might be coming up next, but the respite that the drink gave was short-lived. I still struggle with this deep sense of insecurity and feelings of impending doom, but now I am less fearful about the future. These feelings are less frequent and I have been learning to take a stand against their intrusions into my mind.

I am now open to the idea that rather than living under the shadow of impending doom I can live under the umbrella of providence that is just as able to bring blessing and good things into my life. I now believe that good things can come to me.

6.7 Higher Power

For many years I had two higher powers in the form of two spirits wrestling for control of my life. At times the Spirit of God seemed to be winning but it was a constant wrestling match as the alcoholic spirit and the Spirit of God vied for supremacy.

I knew that God didn't want me to drink but I just couldn't put it down. Actually, I didn't want to as my will was attached to it with superglue. I just couldn't say goodbye to alcohol as I could not imagine any sort of life worth living without it.

No matter how long I went without it the opportune time would come and I would always pick up again. It wasn't until I got to the end of myself that I was able to let go and let God do what I couldn't do for myself.

I had to be willing to say that I wanted this entity to be removed from me so that I could find deliverance from its grip. It had hold of me and I had hold of it. I needed to let go and as I did so the miracle was that it let go of me. It loosened its grip enough for me to pull away and break free.

Of course, it is still waiting with its arm held out to me offering me a helping hand. Today, my higher power is God and not alcohol. He is the one that I cling to and hold onto now. It is God's power that is now being demonstrated in my life as I stay sober for yet another day.

That's the God of my understanding, my higher power, keeping me sober, keeping me safe.

6.8 Turn It Over

Deciding to go to Alcoholics Anonymous was for me an admission of powerlessness. By walking through that door, I was turning the whole alcohol problem over to a power greater than myself. I'd tried everything and I couldn't sort it out. I just couldn't put the drink down and enjoy life.

Since turning my alcohol problem over I am learning to turn many other problems over instead of coming at them head on using my willpower. Step by step I am being shown what action to take in the practical decisions of life that I used to find difficult or impossible. This is a very practical program of action and my life is getting better as I keep turning it over, whatever it is.

So many things in my life will not yield to a head on assault with will power alone. I need wisdom from above and I have to recognise that there are situations where it is difficult or impossible for me to know the way ahead.

All I can do it turn it over to the one who know everything and leave it with him until such time as I get further instructions.

6.9 Bullied

Growing up in an alcoholic home meant that I just got used to being around bullying behaviour. Bullying was normal and as a child, I accepted it as the norm.

I went to a rough primary school when I was five years old and I was bullied. As a teenager in another type of tough school, I again experienced bullying. Later in friendships and in the work-place I found myself being bullied.

At the time I didn't recognise it but as I started to come out of the alcoholic world, I became aware of just how much of a target for bullying I had become. It was almost as if I had a neon sign flashing on my forehead saying 'bully me'.

Drinking locked me into bullying and abusive relationships and whilst I still find myself falling prey to bullies, in recovery, I am learning to protect myself and I am less prone to suffer at the hands of life's bullies.

6.10 Obsession

Some music and songs work like worms in my head and the more they get into my mind the harder they are to get rid of. My obsession with alcohol was like a worm in my head dominating my thoughts and feelings with the persistent idea of and desire for a drink.

The word obsession comes from the word 'besiege' and that describes my condition perfectly. My mind would be besieged by the persistent thought of a drink as well as the impulse to act out on it.

It was a compulsive preoccupation that would get me fixated on the idea of taking a drink even when I didn't want to. Like the worm in the head, it was involuntary and continuous.

Thankfully the obsession has lifted and as long as I don't reactivate it by taking a drink all is well.

6.11 Vulnerability

Drinking resulted in my becoming vulnerable to abuse, manipulation, deception and control. I didn't have to be drunk to be vulnerable although my intoxication did put me in some dangerous situations. Some people seemed to latch onto my weakness caused by alcoholism and they used it for their own advantage.

Looking back, I can see how people used fear to dominate and manipulate me into doing things for them that were not right. I could not seem to say 'no' and would be pushed into hastily agreeing to things that I should never have agreed to. This caused me a lot of stress as I felt torn on the inside between what I knew to be right and the wrong action that I was taking because I was being manipulated and used.

My drinking turned me into a vulnerable person and even now in recovery, I find myself in situations where I am being bullied, manipulated or deceived without realising it. In sobriety I need to take care, to recognise that I attract bullies and that I am still vulnerable to their abuse.

6.12 Change

One of the best things about recovery is that I have changed and that I am continuing to change for the better. Instead of my life being on hold and stuck in many different negative patterns of thinking and living I am now experiencing real change. It's fantastic to be able to change and to be able to recognise that I am not like I was anymore. I have changed and I am not the same person that I was before I came into recovery.

There are so many negative things that I have been able to leave behind and so many positive things that are coming into my life now. My whole operating system has been replaced as I have worked the program of recovery that has been given to me.

I no longer beat myself up about the past because through the program I have put the past to bed and I am now living in the present. I no longer need to live in guilt and shame because I have moved on from the negative things that defined my life before recovery.

I am living a new life and I am experiencing the freedom of being able to change one day at a time.

6.13 The Gift of Recovery

I can so easily forget that my recovery from alcoholism is a gift and not a right. It is given by the grace of God and it is given one day at a time. When people ask me how I stopped drinking I have to be honest and say that I don't really know. There was an element of miracle about it and it wasn't something that I had worked for.

My only contribution was to take it to such an extreme that I couldn't break free without the intervention of a higher power. The danger for me is that I can forget that recovery is a gift and I can begin to think that it's all in my power and under my control. The great illusion of control is always waiting in the wings to take over and lead me back out from under the gift of recovery.

The word grace means gift and I know that it is by the grace of God that I have been given the gift of recovery. I do not want to squander this precious gift and I know that the way to keep it is to give it away.

The more I give recovery away the more recovery I receive. There is no limit to the grace of God.

6.14 Taking Down Barriers

What I am really doing as I work on removing my defects of character in my recovery program is the taking down of the barriers that I have put up between me and God. The result of my alcoholic behaviours and alcoholic thinking was that my wilfulness and its actions became a barrier between myself and God.

I wanted God in my life but I did not want God interfering too much, especially in my drinking life, so I needed to keep him at a distance. I wanted to keep my independence and the only way I could do that was to separate myself from God.

A big part of the foundational work that I have been doing in recovery is clearing away the debris that has formed into a barrier between myself and God. Each day in prayer and meditation, I am seeking to remove more barriers and clear the road between myself and my God. As I take down my barriers, I am finding that there are no barriers on his side. All the blockages and obstacles are on my side as God has already cleared the path on his end.

The door will open if I will only clear the debris on my side that is blocking it from opening properly. It tends to open a bit and then I push some obstacle against it that slams it closed again. The work I am doing in recovery is aimed at keeping the door open so that I don't have to live separated from my higher power who constantly holds me in recovery.

6.15 The Booze Bank

Drinking involved heavy investment, not in a savings account with the bank, but in a constant stream of bottles into the bottle bank. Every week I would save up all the empty bottles and put them in the bottle bank. Over the years I invested heavily in alcohol and all I had to show for it was empties in the booze bottle bank.

I recently stayed at an expensive hotel but my luxury suite was next to the car park where the bottle bank was situated. It was a wealthy place and I was intrigued as a stream of Bentley and Proche cars qued up so that their smartly dressed occupants could noisily deposit huge quantities of empty bottles in the glass recycling bank. I guess they were getting rid of the evidence and I wondered how many of them were pondering the excessive amounts of expensive vintages they were consuming?

A lot of people never even get their bottles or cans to the recycling centre or bottle bank. When I used to run, I was always intrigued by the bundles of empty cans tied up in plastic bags that had been thrown into the hedgerows. It is amazing the way that empty bottles and cans mount up providing unwanted evidence of overall alcohol consumption which is why the bottle bank is such an important feature of life even for the upper-class drinker.

I guess this is what makes the switch to wine boxes such an attractive move as they are easier to get rid of and also helpful in terms of obscuring true levels of overall consumption from ones self as well as from others.

6.16 More Tea Vicar

When I first came off alcohol, I was drinking endless cups of tea and coffee to quench my thirst. I was still very thirsty and transferred my thirst for alcohol onto tea and coffee.

As an alcoholic I find the idea of moderation to be difficult as I seem to have an 'all or nothing' approach to everything. I have had to learn to moderate my coffee intake as I have found myself overdosing on it and ending up with stomach pains or caffeine jitters.

My capacity for endless cups of tea has proved to be a significant plus in terms of my career as a vicar. I can visit a number of homes in succession and have a mug of tea in each of them without ill effect. I just no longer take up the offer of the sherry!

I also love the fact that all the recovery meetings start with a cup of tea or coffee and often a biscuit. It might sound trivial but we are still ex-drinkers and our fellowship grows as we are able to get together to eat, to drink and to share our experience, strength and hope.

I am very thankful that my decision to quit alcohol has coincided with the rise of the coffee shop culture that has provided me with an alternative social drinking location to replace the pub.

6.17 An Alcoholic Mind

When I first heard people in recovery talking about an alcoholic mind, I thought that it was a bit far-fetched. Is there really such a thing as an alcoholic mind? At first, I couldn't accept this idea and I thought it was a bit over the top. I now recognise that I really do have an alcoholic mind and I think in a way that is consistent with the way that other alcoholics think.

How do I know this? The answer is that I have now listened to hundreds of hours of other alcoholics sharing their experience of this disease and I can see that I have many of the common mental twists and turns that are peculiar to alcoholics.

The most obvious one is that I have no mental defence against the first drink. Before I came into recovery no amount of self-knowledge or willpower could help me from picking up the first drink.

I have also discovered that my alcoholic mentality reaches way beyond drinking and into many other areas of my life where my thinking is distorted by my alcoholic mind.

One of the advantages of having friends in recovery is that I can check up on my best thinking with them so that I don't act out of the distorted perspective that comes with my alcoholic mindset.

6.18 Beautiful Scars

I have been listening to a gospel song called 'Beautiful Scars' and it is bringing tears to my eyes. When we come into recovery from alcohol addiction, we bear the marks of pain in the form of emotional and physical scars.

Some of us have scars from self-harm or from physical wounds inflicted by others. We have been abused by those who have taken advantage of our addiction and we carry those scars.

In recovery, I am finding that there is a beauty in my scars which are tokens of my experience that can be turned around and used to help other people out of the prison of addiction. I am comforted by the fact that even Jesus showed people the wounds in his hands, his feet and his side. They were proof, not only of his suffering but also his victory and the new kind of life that he was living.

In recovery, my scars take on a new meaning and a new beauty as I live a new and different life from the one that was just bringing pain and death to everything meaningful.

6.19 A Spiritual Program

I have come to see that the spiritual comes before the material and my recovery from alcoholism has its roots in the realm of the spirit. I am convinced that behind my constant thirst for alcohol was an intense spiritual thirst for God. I am thirsty for something and someone other than what or who I can find in this world. I have had a restless spirit that can't find satisfaction in this world. I need something else, something deeper than what I experience in ordinary life.

I remember thinking to myself, is this it? Is this all there is? There must be more to life than this? Alcohol provided some temporary relief but it never took away my thirst and just quenched my spirit leaving me more frustrated than ever.

I see my alcoholism as a disease of the spirit as well as a disease of body and mind. When I feed my spirit and invest in my spiritual life, I find that healing comes to my soul and my thirst for alcohol is relieved.

6.20 This Too Shall Pass

This slogan that I first saw on the wall of a recovery meeting room has been invaluable as I have had to learn to sit with my feelings instead of suppressing them. Alcoholism in my home meant that I could not express my emotions and I grew up lacking in emotional intelligence.

Until coming into recovery I had not learned to identify, sit with, and process my feelings. I could not untangle my feelings or make sense of them, so I just 'stuffed' them and shoved them down. For a long time, alcohol provided a way of keeping my feelings at bay but when I quit drinking these long-suppressed feelings started to manifest and I didn't know how to process them.

This slogan helped me because it enabled me to learn that no matter how uncomfortable I was feeling, I could be reassured that it was not going to last forever. I have learned that feelings come and go so that however intense they may be, they will not last long.

For no obvious reason, I regularly walk into a mist of fear that envelops me to such an extent that I feel that it will never go. At such times I remind myself that this too shall pass, if I just allow myself to feel it and press on with doing what I am meant to be doing, then I will be alright.

6.21 Triggers

I have found it helpful to notice when I am disturbed by some event or happening in my life and to ask myself what is going on. It could be something that somebody says, maybe an email or something in the media. I am learning not to ignore these triggers but to take note of them and to seek to understand what they are saying to me about growth and change.

I recently found myself gripped and worried by something that was shared in a meeting. It triggered my fear for a loved one and what I realised when I looked at this fear was that I was trying to control their life and keep them safe in a way that was impossible. Their life was outside and beyond my control and I realised that I was acting out of my fear for them as well as fear for myself. My protective behaviour was not going to make any difference and it could even have made the situation worse.

It made me realise afresh that I cannot change other people but I can change myself and my own behaviour. It reinforced the truth that I am not God and I can't control how other people live their lives, so I have to let go and let God.

This insight came from my own reflection on this single trigger event that before coming into recovery I would most likely have just avoided thinking about.

6.22 Responding or Reacting

My high levels of fear combined with my desire to please people means that I have a tendency to react instead of responding to requests or demands.

Today I received an email and my inner urge was to react and send an immediate reply. My need to please was so strong and combined with my insecurity and fear I felt a compulsion to act and to act now. Everything in me wanted to take immediate action but I am learning to stop and to resist the temptation to react.

I realise how I have been acting out of fear and the desire to please people instead of responding calmly after a time of reflection to think about what might be the best course of action. In fact, I don't need to give an immediate response at all and it will be better if I ask my higher power to give me wisdom and show me the way forward. I am now putting the matter on hold to give myself time to think and to respond well if I even decide to respond at all.

Reacting from a desire to please has cost me dearly in the past as I have hastily agreed to things that I should never have agreed to. I have felt a false pressure and an irrational need to please by saying yes when the answer should have been to say let's think about it or even no.

6.23 Compromised Faith

I had spiritual awakenings and many profound spiritual experiences before I came into recovery. These experiences and spiritual awakenings that came to me through my faith did enable me to cut down on my drinking but not to stop entirely. My faith and the lifestyle that developed from it had the effect of putting the brakes on my drinking, but this did not eliminate my underlying alcoholism.

Like shingles, it lay dormant in me until the opportune time came for it to manifest its true grip on me. As my drinking picked up momentum in mid-life it led me increasingly into a lifestyle that was in conflict with my beliefs. My drinking compromised my faith and at one point nearly destroyed it as I began to doubt everything that I had been taught about God.

Drinking took away my confidence in God to the point where I began to doubt his existence. I was internally conflicted as the compulsion to drink battled it out with my beliefs. I knew it was wrong for me to drink and that God didn't want me to, but I just couldn't stop.

Although I felt that I should have been able to find release from the bondage to alcohol through my faith I could not. Recovery meetings have shown me how to access my faith in a way that works when it comes to gaining victory over alcohol addiction.

My faith and my experience of God is no longer being undermined and compromised by the compulsion to drink alcohol.

6.24 Personality Change

A friend of mine was telling me how she can see the change that takes place in her alcoholic mother after her mum takes just a few sips of wine. To most people that might seem a bit far-fetched but to me as a recovering alcoholic it makes a lot of sense.

When I used to take in even just a small amount of alcohol something happened to me. I remember being at a dinner party where I felt quite awkward and ill at ease but after just a few mouthfuls of wine I felt invigorated and all my fears vanished as I became vocal and animated. There was a sense in which I became another person as I underwent a personality change as a result of drinking alcohol.

Many other alcoholics out there also experience this personality change and it can have some pretty dire consequences. Fights, stabbings, arguments and some really ugly behaviour can emerge from a normally placid and quiet person who undergoes a personality change after taking even just a few drinks.

6.25 Blind Drunk

If you had said to me when I was drinking that I was putting myself and my family in danger by going to the pub after work, I would have said you were crazy. What I realise now is that I was blind to the dangers and risks that I was taking when I was drinking.

Once I took a drink my normal sense of danger was greatly reduced and my chances of risky behaviour increased. How easy it would have been to have got arrested for drink driving and to have lost my livelihood, home and reputation as a result.

The implications would have been really catastrophic for my wife and children as they would through no fault of their own found themselves homeless and without an income because of their father's idiotic behaviour caused by his drinking.

I was blind to all these things when I was drinking and I selfishly put a lot of other people lives at risk in the process. Thankfully I don't do this anymore.

6.26 Sneaking Drinks

At times in my drinking, my alcoholic habit involved getting as many drinks down my throat as I could whilst trying to avoid alerting anyone else to the fact that this is what I was doing. It demanded multiple forms of deception as I tried to figure out ways to take on board more alcohol.

There are of course many tried and tested methods of sneaking drinks like having several bottles on the go at the same time with one on the table and another hidden nearby. Drinks can be sneaked at all times and in all places. Miniatures still seem to be a popular way to get in a few cheeky ones without arousing too much suspicion, as these smaller bottles can be easily secreted in cases, bags and jacket pockets.

In recovery, it is such a relief not to have to engage in this ridiculous game of hide and seek with alcohol.

Thank God that there is no more deception, guilt and fear of discovery in the endless game of sneaking drinks.

6.27 Steady

I asked an alcoholic barman friend of mine how his drinking was going and he said 'steady'. I knew exactly what he meant. He was keeping himself topped up but not pushing himself into full-on drunkenness. I guess there was some form of control in this but eventually, his drinking, like mine, got out of control and ultimately led to him taking his own life just before his fiftieth birthday.

People imagine that if you are an alcoholic, you are more or less insanely drunk all of the time but this is not so. Many alcoholics achieve some sort of balance so that they are constantly in a partially anesthetised state but not incapacitated.

Functioning alcoholics often go for years keeping their intake reasonably steady most of the time. The problem is that increased tolerance and the desire for more keeps pushing alcoholic drinkers further on into the more advanced stages of the disease where normal functioning becomes almost impossible.

6.28 Moments of Perception

One of the things that has happened to me since coming into recovery is that I get moments of perception where I can see things much more clearly. I can see and understand things that I didn't notice or comprehend before.

I can't control this flow of perception and some days or even weeks there seems to be little or none. But at other times my mind is opened up in new ways so that I can see perceive and experience life differently.

Sometimes a perceptive thought just flashes across my mind or I get the solution to a difficult problem for which I previously had no answer. At other times these moments of perception provide an insight into a truth that has been previously hidden from my view.

These revelations make life more interesting and open up a new sense of discovery and wonder about this amazing world of which I am just the tiniest part.

Perhaps these moments of perception were always there but alcohol dulled my senses and cut me off from my childhood sense of awe and wonder.

6.29 Learning to Listen

It is only since coming into recovery that I have begun to learn to listen. Not so long ago my son stopped me in the kitchen and said 'dad you're listening to me.' I was shocked because I realised that what this comment meant was that for a lot of his life, I had not been giving him the attention he needed. I had been absorbed in my own world and consumed with my self-centred thinking so that my son never felt that he was being listened to.

Now I try to give him my maximum attention when he is speaking to me and sharing his life with me. In recovery, as I have heard other people telling their stories I have been learning to listen and that attentiveness has spread to my own family and beyond. Before I just could not listen without butting in or putting 'my oar in.'

Now I am learning to just 'shut it' and listen. I still find it difficult but I know how much I value it when I feel that I have been listened to.

I am realising that the simple act of listening to another person is a free gift that I can give away to all who come across my path in life.

6.30 Feeling Alcoholic

I used to go to a recovery meeting where a man would regularly say that he was feeling really alcoholic. This perplexed me and I found myself wondering what he meant. Now that I have been in recovery a while, I have a much better understanding of what he was saying.

I experience days where I feel really alcoholic without the involvement of alcohol. Today I have been struggling with a set of feelings and a mindset that I would label as alcoholic. I feel on-edge, restless, jumpy, unable to settle on any particular task or to fully concentrate on anything. I am experiencing a lot of negative thoughts especially about my life and my imagined future. My vision is darkened by projections of negative and imaginary circumstances where everything is falling apart. I am worried about not being up to the challenges ahead of me and I don't believe that I will be able to cope with this bleak imaginary future that is playing out in my mind.

At this moment I feel like a failure with my head constantly reinforcing that idea that I am not good enough and that I might as well just give up.

I know that this cloudy emotional weather will blow over and tomorrow I may well be on top of the world, but today I am suffering from the disease of alcoholism.

Today I am feeling really alcoholic, but I have learned in recovery that I will not be feeling like this for long.

July

7.1 The Prime Suspect

What happened to me when I came into recovery was that I realised that rather than being the solution to my problems, alcohol was the cause. When I look back at the problems and difficulties that I was experiencing at the time I can now see that the great majority of them had their roots in alcoholic drinking. When I was drinking, I could not see clearly enough to recognise that alcohol was the common denominator in the trouble that I was having with doing life.

Recovery started as I began to realise that alcohol was the prime suspect in all my troubles with living. Alcohol had pretended to be my friend but behind the scenes, it was pulling me to pieces. Alcohol was destroying me whilst masquerading as a faithful colleague who flattered me and told me lies.

Finally, I got suspicious and these suspicions were confirmed in the rooms of recovery as I realised that I was not the only one who had been betrayed by alcohol. Alcohol is a cunning foe that for many years pretended to be my friend whilst doing everything it could behind the scenes to ruin my life and bring me down.

7.2 Victims No More

I am no longer a victim of alcohol. I have agency and I am free from the bondage of alcoholic drinking. I am no longer at the beck and call of alcohol. I am no longer its slave and I am no longer a victim of its punishing regime. I no longer have to live a life that is less than God intended for me.

At last, I can now live out the life that God has given me. I am no longer living in alcohol-induced shame and guilt. I can get on with my life and pursue the vision that God has given me for the future without being held back by alcoholic fear.

I am now living one life not two. I have no other agenda other than living out the will and purposes of God for the rest of my life. I am free to be the person I was created to be and I thank God that I don't have to live life as a victim anymore.

7.3 Alcohol Wants Me Dead

It might seem an extreme thing to say that alcohol wants me dead, but this is the truth. Alcohol wants me to hang, but now that I have rumbled it, I can see all the dirty tricks that it has played on me.

Alcohol wants me dead; it hates me and will do anything it can to get me out of its way. Alcohol wants to destroy my life and the lives of all around me. Alcohol is a ruthless killer who will stop at nothing to destroy its victim.

I am now under no illusions; every possible underhanded and deceptive tactic is in the hands of this formidable foe. I can never afford to underestimate this evil and manipulative power who will use anything and anyone to get hold of me and destroy me.

Just because I have escaped its grip alcohol has not forgotten me and is waiting to take any opportunity that it can to take me down. I have to take every precaution that I can to make sure that I am well beyond the reach of alcohol and I pray for constant protection against this ever-present enemy.

7.4 Taking a Trip

I once took half a tab of LSD in a bar in the city. I vaguely remember feeling about thirty feet tall and I have dim recollections of the events in the following hours.

It reminds me that particularly near the end of my drinking I knew that when I took a drink, I didn't really know what was going to happen or how it was going to end. I was taking a trip but I didn't know the destination.

Although I didn't realise it at the time the act of taking the first drink was for me like handing over control of my life to a higher power. I was putting my life in the hands of a spirit who was promising me a good time.

It is true that alcohol gave me many good times and I had a lot of fun with it. However, near the end of my drinking, I don't remember it being so much fun anymore. It was all a bit of a chore and it was causing me a lot of trouble. Hangovers, headaches, depression, negativity and a sense of lostness.

I felt guilty, ashamed and a fraud. I was meant to be and wanted to be a holy man but my drinking was taking me on a one-way trip to an early grave.

7.5 The Obsession to Drink

The obsession to drink left me when I came into recovery. It just lifted off me so that I no longer found myself thinking obsessively about my next drink. I can't explain it and it is a miracle because all I did was act on the thought that I need to get help for my drinking. I gave up trying to use my own wisdom and understanding to solve the mystery of my obsessive use of alcohol.

Whilst I experienced some effects of physical withdrawal, I was spared the mental craving and obsessive thinking about my next drink. I stopped planning to drink and gave in to the idea that one day at a time I wasn't going to pick up a drink.

I suppose I became as obsessed with not drinking as I had been with drinking. Very quickly I got my life back and there was no more obsessive thinking about alcohol. I did get obsessive with my studies but that was a lot better than the drinking.

In time I have become less obsessive about everything as the obsession with drink has been removed.

7.6 Reading Rock Festival

In 1974 I found myself at what was known then as the 'Reading Rock Festival.' It was a far cry from the corporately sponsored and stylised 'glamping' events of today. The place was awash with drugs. There was quite a lot of acid but for most of us, it was just Afghan black and alcohol as we tried to avoid the constant rain of empty bottles that people threw at each other across the muddy site.

The prog-rock band 'YES' were headlining on the main stage and it was a psychedelic paradise, or a drink and drugs hell, depending on how you look at it.

I'm glad I went because I have witnessed first-hand the reality behind hippy festival nostalgia with the degradation and abuse that lay just below the surface of what we considered 'cool.'

I suppose it was one of the more interesting places that alcohol took me in my early years.

7.7 Detoxification

Detoxification can get alcohol out of the body but it can't stop the craving towards intoxication. Detoxification and intoxication cannot exist together and one is always going to win. It has to be a life without alcohol or a life with it and there is no middle ground for me as an alcoholic.

Through taking just one small drink the phenomenon of alcoholic craving is activated so that I have to continue to put the stuff in my body until I can't physically take any more. I guess it must be a bit like a binge eater who has to eat until they are sick.

I have known serious alcoholics who have drunk aftershave to get alcohol back in their system when the craving is on them. Detoxification is but the beginning of the journey into recovery and it is not an easy road, but it is possible. If it were easy then more of us would be on it.

As they say, alcohol is 'cunning, baffling and powerful' but even so it is possible not to go back to a life of intoxication unless I want to.

7.8 Ahead of the Game

I went to a rather expensive prep school in Kent and one of my fellow pupils was a young man called Shane who like me went on to have an interesting relationship with alcohol. He was a very gifted English scholar, a poet, and I guess he was a child prodigy in this respect.

I remember him weeping in the playground over the death of Jimi Hendrix as he walked around clutching his

Hendrix album. We were only twelve years old and I hadn't got much of a clue who Hendrix was, let alone having any familiarity with or liking for his music.

Shane was definitely ahead of the game although he was, even back then, a bit out of it in practical matters. He used to live at the top of our road and I remember him crashing his bike into the flower bed of our front garden after having lost control. Perhaps that was a metaphor for his life.

Years later at the rise of the punk scene and before The Pogues, I met him in the public bar of the Sussex Arms where he offered me a drink. He was on Guinness and maybe that's what's kept him alive through his remarkable and legendary career in music and popular culture.

7.9 The Same Person

I've heard it said that 'the same person will drink again.' What this means is that if I don't change in myself then it's not likely that my relationship with alcohol will change, and if that doesn't change, then I am likely to pick up again.

For years I could never understand why I would always go back to drinking even when I had vowed that I would never drink again. I really meant it at the time but the day would always come, often the next day, and I'd be back on it.

In recovery, I have found that the reason for this was that I had not really changed and therefore my behaviours were not going to change.

I now live a life of positive and intentional recovery and I am experiencing deep personal change as I submit to the simple program that I have been given. It really works and I know that because something has happened to me deep down inside so that I no longer have a desire or craving to drink.

I am not the same person that I was and I now feel that I have every chance of ongoing recovery and positive change in my life.

7.10 Character

My alcoholic life was not good for my character as it allowed my character defects to go unchecked and gain more ground in my life. Fear, pride, insecurity, people-pleasing, impressing people, selfishness, impulsiveness, inappropriate behaviour and a lack of self-control all had the opportunity to flourish under the umbrella of a drinking life.

It has only been in the recovery program that I have gradually been able to identify my character defects as the fog of alcoholism has lifted. I realise that my drinking resulted in a form of arrested development that prevented me from growing up as I should have done. Alcohol blinded me and prevented me from seeing myself as I really was.

Now I can see my personal defects much more clearly and with the help of others in recovery as well as the program I have been able to eliminate some of my more destructive character defects. The good thing is that this makes life so much easier as I am not creating chaos or trouble for myself or anyone else. I am enjoying the challenge of working on my character defects with the help of my God. It's a lifetime project but a fascinating one and a really positive thing to do.

As I grow older, I want to be getting better rather than worse as a person. I want to be more useful to God and to the people around me. I want to be a good, helpful and fun person to be around. I want to make a positive impact on my world and I am far more likely to do this if I am not hauling around a bag full of character defects.

7.11 My Reward

For a long time, alcohol was my reward at the weekend or at the end of a day's work. I felt that I deserved a drink and it gave me something to aim for during the day or as the weekend approached.

Drinking was something that I always looked forward to and I looked at the next opportunity to drink as my reward. I don't know what I thought it was a reward for but I certainly felt that I was entitled to it and that somehow, I had earned the right to drink.

This reward mentality is still part of my thinking so these days I have to find legitimate and reasonably healthy ways to reward myself. Cups of tea, coffees, biscuits, cakes, buns, crisps and chocolate have taken the place of Guinness and wine.

Because I am sober and not hungover, I can reward myself by enjoying some of the simple pleasures in life such as a walk in the country or a stroll along the beach. I now have some money in my pocket so I can also reward myself with some nice things that bring me more lasting pleasure like a new watch or a new pair of sunglasses.

7.12 The Top Shelf

I thank God for my weak stomach that made it almost impossible for me to drink spirits. This meant that when drinking I mostly stuck with beer and wine and avoided the top shelf. I could not keep vodka down but I could just about stomach small quantities of Jameson's Irish Whisky or dark rum.

Like many of my drinking friends, I ended up on a steady diet of draught Guinness which I regard as the methadone of alcoholic drinks. Guinness had a particular effect on me that sort of numbed my brain and sedated me. I used little bottles of strong lager as a catalyst and wine provided the delivery vehicle for alcohol when I was full up with beer.

This was the simple chemistry set that enabled me to enjoy drinking for many years. I'm sure that if I had been able to stomach it, I would have been at the top shelf and my demise would have been much swifter.

7.13 Functioning Alcoholic

I was what people call a functioning alcoholic in the sense that I still had a job, a family, a car, a house and a wife. However, when I finally arrived in recovery, I was struggling in all of these areas of life.

Since my teenage years, I had used alcohol as a way of getting by and alcohol had served as a crutch that helped me through things that I found difficult. Although I was functioning outwardly, on the inside I was struggling with low mood, fear, anxiety and paranoia.

Somehow, I kept going but if I had not gone to a recovery meeting and accepted help, I am sure that my world would have collapsed around me. I was on a precipice but thank God I didn't go over the top.

I am now functioning much better due to the power of the program and the power of God behind it. I guess I can now call myself a functioning recovering alcoholic.

7.14 All of It

My God was pleased to step in and take over my alcohol problem when I finally gave up trying to fix it by myself. I handed it over the day I went to Alcoholics Anonymous looking for a way out of what I came to understand as alcoholism.

What I didn't realise at the time was that God didn't just want my alcohol problem, he wanted me, and he wanted me to hand over all of my life to him. I came to see that every aspect of my life needed to be placed at his disposal and under his authority.

Having acted on this radical proposal my life has been undergoing a never-ending process of change for the better. Everything in my life is being bought under the jurisdiction of a loving God as I understand him.

Slowly but surely my life is being tuned into his wavelength and the signals are getting stronger and stronger. I am being guided further and further into his will and I am finding that as I surrender to his will, my life is working in a way that it never did before.

7.15 Progress

At the height of my drinking, it seemed to me that life was getting worse and worse. It felt like everything was getting darker and the world was closing in on me. I had lost my sense of hope and the future did not look good.

In recovery, I feel very different about my life and I now have my hope back. I can see signs of progress as positive changes take place in my life and I now feel that I have a life that is worth living.

Instead of wanting this life to be over I now want to live longer so that I can help other people who are suffering from this disease. Like many recovering alcoholics I have a special interest in helping other alcoholics to escape from the clutches of alcohol addiction. It is great to feel that my life has a new sense of purpose and that it is progressing and not declining.

I now look forward to the future instead of it filling me with dread, fear and foreboding.

7.16 Defending my Drinking

When I was drinking alcoholically, I used to resent people challenging me about my drinking. I would defend my drinking to the death. My attitude was how dare you criticise my drinking, it's none of your business.

Alcoholism has its own protection mechanism that defends itself at all costs. In family support groups, they say that when it comes to alcoholism you have to realise that you didn't cause it, you can't cure it and you have no control over it.

Alcoholism is siege proof and the only way to defeat it is from within. Like the Trojan Horse, we need recovery programs that work from inside the citadel of alcoholism.

From this bridgehead within the disease itself, victory becomes possible as the recovery programs get to work behind the walls and defences of denial.

7.17 God in the Details

When I handed my will and my life over to the care of God, I had no real idea what this would mean. I was pleased to hand over my drinking but I didn't know how to hand over the rest of my life.

What I am learning is that my higher power is taking care of absolutely everything for me as long as I remain in his will. It is not just the big stuff that I find being taken care of but also the small stuff in my life. The car repair, the doctor's appointment, the gas bill, and many other details of my life are being taken care of in ways that just never used to happen before.

I still have to do things and take action but I am learning to make room for my higher power to move. I no longer feel that I am doing everything on my own and I know that I am not alone anymore.

7.18 Getting Away with It

When I was drinking, I thought that I was getting away with it. In reality I was getting away with nothing as every action had a consequence. I had to keep on drinking because I couldn't face up to the consequences of my behaviour when drinking. The only way I could deal with my conscience was to silence it with yet more booze.

Despite quite a bit of memory loss and black out drinking I can remember many things that didn't go well because of alcohol. I can now see that I didn't get away with anything.

Everything had its price and took its toll on me or those close to me. It is a great relief to be able to be honest and not to have to try and get away with secret alcoholic drinking.

7.19 Things

They say in the rooms of recovery that we have no control over people, places or things. Today the automatic transmission on my car failed and it is going to cost a lot of money to get it fixed.

I am thinking why me? Why my car? Why my transmission? After all, it is not an old car and I have been looking after it. I have been beating myself up about buying the car in the first place wondering if it was the right decision. I am worried about how much it will cost and if the garage will really be able to fix it.

At the end of the day, I have no control over this 'thing'. It is just a 'thing' and I am working on keeping it in its rightful place. This 'thing' has no right to steal my peace, after all, it is just a lump of metal and a load of cogs.

In recovery, I am working on keeping things simple in my life by refusing to accumulate more things. When I wasn't filling the void with alcohol, I used to fill my life by obsessing about the next thing that I was going to buy. I bought some ridiculous and expensive things that served no useful purpose, but at the time I just had to have them. Acquiring and possessing things became important, but like a child with a new Christmas present, it was quickly discarded as I went on the search for the next new thing.

All this was of course chasing the wind and it has left me with a lot of stuff to dispose of. I think I will just have to give it away as the work involved in selling it off is immense. I suppose the positive is that unlike my drinking I do have something to show for this habit even if those things are now unwanted and clogging up my life.

7.20 Anxiety

I am waging war on my anxiety. I am fed up with it controlling my life. My anxiety burns up my emotional and mental energy that could be used for better things. My anxiety takes me out of the present moment and places me into an imaginary future or an imaginary past.

Anxiety drove my drinking by fuelling my need to release the emotional and mental pressure that it put me under. I now refuse to be ruled by anxiety anymore, it is not my higher power.

Bit by bit I am learning to hand over my anxiety to a power greater than myself. This is not an instant fix but a daily process where I am learning to let go of anxiety and allowing it to be replaced with serenity and peace.

7.21 Decisions

One day I made a decision to get help with my alcoholism. I looked up the Alcoholics Anonymous meetings and found one near to where I started my drinking career.

As I sat in the meeting and listened to people sharing their experience of drinking, I immediately identified with what they were saying. I thought I was the only one but I realised that there were lots of drinkers like me who had been through the same sort of experiences with alcohol.

The person who did 'the share' had the same name as me but he also had an almost identical alcohol story to mine.

This decision to go to a meeting followed by the action of showing up changed the whole course of my life. It opened the door for me into a new life of freedom from the obsession to drink.

7.22 Rituals

In my drinking days, I had rituals that centred around alcohol but in recovery, I have rituals that help me stay on track and keep me sober.

My days have bookends as I spend time every morning and sometimes in the evening in what might be called spiritual reflection.

Using a small daily reading book, I try to start the day by setting out in a good orderly direction. I say a couple of short set prayers asking God to direct my thinking and to give me the courage, strength and wisdom to navigate the day ahead.

Before bed, I briefly review the day and reflect on what went well and what needs work. Then I hand it over to God to take care of, leaving it in safe hands whilst I get some sleep.

These simple rituals give me stability and help me to live an enjoyable sober life today.

7.23 Clean House

I grew up in an exceptionally clean house. My mother's co-dependency led her into compulsive cleaning to such an extent that both my brother and I became allergic to bleach.

We were a very clean house outwardly but behind the façade, there was untreated alcoholism that infected our home. As the disease progressed the house just got cleaner and cleaner as my mother tried to deal with my father's behaviour.

Now I like to keep my house clean but what is far more important to me is the type of housecleaning that is talked about in recovery. This is the deep cleaning that takes place day by day as I work and rework my recovery.

Alcoholic ways of being, thinking and living are apt to reappear like dust and dirt in the house. Through attention to the program, I clean house each morning to make sure that I keep on top of the daily influx of resentments, fears, grouches and other alcoholic grime.

7.24 Supply

Any serious drinker knows the importance of securing your supply. This becomes our great mission. The primary purpose of each day is to do whatever is required to secure a supply of alcohol.

I am always amazed at the ability of even the most destitute of us to scrape together enough cash to buy another can or bottle.

Now I put my energies into getting a different kind of supply.

I ask for enough of the grace of God to see me through another sober day and as I do so I find a constant supply of many other good things that make life worth living.

7.25 Stay Out of Your Mind

As an alcoholic, my mind is not always a reliable instrument. Like a faulty aircraft altimeter, it can give false readings that cause me to fly into mountains and crash. I have heard people say 'stay out of your mind there is no adult supervision in there.' I know what they mean because my alcoholic thinking or 'stinking thinking' as some call it can very quickly take me off course.

Trying to think my way out of alcoholic drinking never got me far because it did not result in the required action. I used to believe that if I understood why I drank then I would be able to stop. The problem was that until I stopped drinking I had very little understanding of why I drank. Now having made the decision to stop I am beginning to see some of those reasons.

My action has informed my thinking not the other way round.

7.26 On God's Side

When I was drinking, I knew that for me I was not doing the right thing. I knew that I was flying in the face of God's will and I knew that it was a conscious act of disregard for God's will for my life. I would have all sorts of justifications and arguments up my sleeve about why I had the right to drink but deep down I knew that I was going against the grain.

Drinking is okay for other people but for drinkers like me, alcohol is off-limits. My higher power was very patient with me on this and of course, he allowed me to feel the consequences of not listening to his loving and wise instruction. My will was set against him in this matter and it affected everything else in my dealings with him. It was a running sore and an unhealed wound that although mostly hidden was doing a lot of damage. I always felt that there was something not right in my life when I was drinking. When I took a drink, I had a deep sense that for me it wasn't the right thing to do. In a way that I didn't understand it was off-limits and by taking the drink, I was stepping outside God's will for my life.

Now that I am no longer pursuing drinking, I feel much more in tune and in line with God's will for my life. It's exciting to see how each day unfolds and what God brings to me on a daily basis. I sense more harmony and agreement with the will of God and I am finding that it is a much better way to live.

Each day brings new surprises as I am led and directed in ways that I never was before. I get the sense that I am much more often in the right place at the right time and when I am in the place that God wants me, I am useful to him. I feel guided in a way that I never used to be and I enjoy tuning in my will to God's will as that seems to be when good things happen all around me.

It's an exciting way to live as no two days are the same when I am walking in the will of God.

7.27 Reprogrammed

My drinking habit is still hard wired in me as years of alcoholic drinking programmed me to drink. Even many years after stopping drinking there are certain sets of circumstances that trigger my programming and the thought of a drink comes to me almost automatically.

Wedding receptions, family parties and birthday celebrations all provide cues for my alcoholic pre-programming to spring into life. I have to be really vigilant because on these occasions I feel my social anxiety rising and my automatic response is to reach for a drink.

As well as finding myself with the old feeling of needing a drink, I also notice the tendency to click back into what could be described as a party spirit with all its attendant craziness. At such times I need to focus on being sober and I have to be especially vigilant as these reactions are so deeply grooved within me. I am still programmed to want to party and that involves drinking as these two things are inseparably joined in my psyche.

A little while ago I accidentally took some wrong turnings on the way to a store and ended up outside a music pub just at the time the bands were unloading their gear. Everything in me wanted to go in there and get stuck in. It was magnetic in its attraction and although I managed to drive away, I longed to go back.

There are occasions like this when my programming is set in motion and it often takes me by surprise. I have good defences against the first drink now but incidents like this alert me to the dangers of complacency in drinking situations.

Some alcoholics tell me that it just doesn't bother them anymore and for the most part, I am not affected. But just occasionally something sets in motion my pre-programming so that I find myself contemplating the thought of a drink.

I don't think I will ever be immune from these automatic impulses but thankfully I have now hardwired and programmed a significant amount of recovery strategies and defensive thinking, which so far, has always cut in and shut down my alcoholic pre-programming.

I guess that I have been partially but not totally reprogrammed.

7.28 Thinking in Extremes

As an alcoholic, I have come to recognise that I have been plagued by all or nothing thinking. This type of mentality was foundational to my wild and excessive drinking. Like many others caught up in alcohol addiction, I could not see the point in having just one drink. Even a few drinks seemed pretty futile to me because I always wanted to go all out until I was unconscious. Knock out drinking was the name of the game for me because if I started, I just had to finish the job. For many years I would prefer not to drink at all rather than have one drink, as just having one drink seemed pointless to me.

This all or nothing thinking was not confined to drinking as whatever I did had to be full on or not at all. I couldn't just go to church I had to become a priest. I couldn't just do some running it has to be marathon running. My whole way of thinking and living was dominated by extremes.

In recovery, I have had to learn to avoid all or nothing thinking. I see this type of all or nothing thinking as being part of my compulsive and impulsive nature. Once I get an obsessive thought in my mind it's difficult to put the brakes on it as it tends to dominate my thinking until I act on it.

I can buy far too many of something and then months later wonder why I bought so many of those things that I now don't know what to do with. I have always found the idea of moderation very difficult to grasp hold of. Moderation never appealed to me before as I thought it showed a lack of passion and commitment.

However, I am slowly learning to avoid extreme behaviour and the extreme thinking behind it. I am starting to embrace the notion of moderation as a possible solution to some of life's situations.

The only place that moderation doesn't work for me is with drinking because when it comes to alcohol it still is all or nothing and I am sticking with the nothing.

7.29 Tormenting Myself

I still engage in the process of tormenting myself with past mistakes or future worries. I find that I am torturing myself with apocalyptic visions of the future. Where will I end up and what will happen to me? I get plagued by these tormenting thoughts and negative projections about the future. I still find myself slipping so naturally into these old patterns of thinking.

Today as I unlocked the front door and looked at the post, I began to wonder what bad news was going to come through these letters and what problems or disasters of the day I would need to be ready for. This is not a healthy attitude to life and betrays my alcoholic mind.

In recovery, I now know the importance of developing positive expectancy about the future. A friend of mine keeps reassuring me that the best is yet to come, but as an alcoholic, I always think that things are getting worse and will decline.

When I was drinking, I could always see the things in the future that I thought were bound to go wrong. Of course, when I was drinking things did go wrong, but nowadays, I am learning to expect better and to have the faith that God has better things in store for me than I have ever had before.

Someone told me that the way to be happy as you get older is to expect better things right up to the end of your life. The most encouraging people I know are the ones who are always expecting better. They see the future as a world of opportunity rather than a theatre of gloom and impending tragedy.

I am slowly crawling out of my inherited alcoholic gloom as I take hold of an attitude of positive expectancy towards my life both now and in the future.

7.30 The Challenge to Change

One of the hardest things about giving up alcohol is facing up to change. As long as I was drinking, I could always hide from or put off changing for as long as possible. I just don't like change and I want things to stay exactly the way they are.

Changing from being a drinker to a non-drinker seemed at the time to be the biggest decision that I had ever made. I could not imagine life without drink, and therefore the change was more than I could contemplate, which is why I put it off for so long.

I still hold onto things much longer than I should do and I know the reason why. It's because I feel that I need the security that they bring me. I find a deep resistance to letting go of people, places or things. I hold on to them for dear life because they provide me with a sense of security, but I know that holding onto them for too long causes me problems.

I need to change, I need to move on, and I need to let go, but it is so hard for me to do this. Things are changing faster than ever and I am having to get used to this constant challenge to change in every area of my life.

I am also having to acknowledge that whilst I don't like some of the changes, some of them actually make life better for me. I recently had to change my car and I could not let go of the old one. In fact, it's still on the driveway of my house and eventually, I will have to call the scrap dealer to take it away. However, despite my reluctance to change, I am now enjoying the new car which is a lot easier to drive and makes my daily life much less hard work.

The challenge to change is all around me and I pray for the courage to make the changes that I need to make in my life.

7.31 Recovery First

As the days become years in recovery, I have to remember that without my sobriety everything is lost. My whole life is now built on the firm foundation of a non-drinking life, so keeping that foundation well maintained is a priority. This means putting recovery first in my life, and of course, this is a challenge as life takes off and gets busy.

I was recently asked if I would like a new job. It was a very good, challenging and interesting one. It was certainly a good career move but as I reflected on it, I began to see that if I took the job there would be very little if any time or energy left over for anything else including my recovery meetings and commitments. I realised that if I took the job, I could easily end up compromising or even jeopardising my ongoing recovery. As I thought it through, I realised that if I took such a position, I could even end up relapsing and then all would be lost.

I guess it's about knowing my limits and having the common sense to realise when I am overreaching myself and putting my recovery in danger. I have to accept that in a way I do have to live with limits like anyone with a difficult disease, albeit one that is in remission.

Most of the time it doesn't affect me as long as I remember that my recovery always has to be the priority and as long as I put my recovery first, I will be alright.

August

8.1 People without a Program

Even if we are living a program of recovery we have to live with people without a program and this can be frustrating. The insights and the growing sense of self-awareness, not to mention sensitivity to the spirit may well not be available to them.

A friend of mine calls these people who seem to stand in our path of progress, grace growers. They are placed in our way so that we can learn to develop and grow spiritual muscle as they stretch the quality and depth of our recovery. They haven't done the work, they have no reason to, but we are doing the work and we have good reason to.

I have to keep sober so I have to work my program if I want to keep moving forward and not fall back into the abyss of alcoholism. How many of us would have taken up this new way of life if we could have avoided it?

We are incentivised, we have a program, we are the lucky ones.

8.2 Powerlessness

I really didn't want to accept the idea that I am powerless over alcohol. Why should I allow alcohol to have that much power over me?

Surely, I have some control and power over it, after all it's me who opens the bottles and drinks it? This seems logical but alcoholism is not logical.

We can understand aspects of it but it defies understanding and illudes that much sought after medical holy grail of a cure.

I started to admit my powerlessness the day I walked into a recovery meeting and listened to the people sharing. Gradually I let go of my old idea that I have any power over alcohol.

Alcohol has power over me and that is why I need the program.

8.3 First Things First

My recovery from alcoholism has accelerated or stalled depending on the priority that I have given it in my life. Of course, initially, my recovery took off when I decided to put the program into first place in my life. I prioritised meeting over all other activities including work.

When I took my foot off the gas and let other things take over my progress slowed and almost stalled at times. It wasn't until recently when I decided to put this God-given program in absolute first place that I started to get the deep recovery that I had been looking for.

Up until this time I was holding something back and could not quite give myself fully to the process. However, now that I really am putting recovery first, I have been able to figure out other priorities in my life.

I had always struggled to know what to do first, what to do next and when. I would get very confused and conflicted about my priorities especially as I was trying to keep everybody happy. This meant that I found it difficult to make even simple decisions.

Putting first things first has meant that I am learning to figure out what I should be doing next and what I can leave to another time or another day. As long as I put recovery first, I find that everything else seems to eventually find its rightful place in my life.

One of the definitions of God that I have heard in the rooms is good orderly direction and I certainly have gained some of that these days.

8.4 Go to a Meeting

The brilliant thing about belonging to Alcoholics Anonymous is that there is always a meeting going on somewhere at any time of the day or night. I can join meetings all over the globe if I want to.

Connecting with a meeting is a great tonic when things are difficult and alongside phoning a sponsor it is one of the main lifelines in recovery.

We can't do this on our own, we need each other and the meetings provide that essential contact that keeps us on the rails.

I remember the sense of relief that I experienced the day I realised that whatever was going on in my life, however difficult, I could always go to a meeting.

People talk about the psychic change that they experience through attending meetings and I know what they mean. I can arrive in a real state and leave in a much better frame of mind.

Meetings are rarely boring and if I'm bored it's generally me and not the meeting that's to blame.

I love going to recovery meetings.

8.5 Inside Out

Something deep inside of me used to resist and reject the whole idea of discipline. I was familiar with external discipline having been brought up in a military home and then a strict boarding school, but what I lacked was a personal and inner discipline.

My discipline had been imposed and it was outside in. What I discovered in recovery was that I needed to live from the inside out and that internally generated inner discipline is far more powerful.

I now keep the kitchen clean and tidy not because I have to but because I want to. I now keep the laundry up to date because I want to and enjoy the sense of being on top of domestic life.

I do my job properly and well because I want to not just because I have to. It's the program that has taught me this and God by his grace has given me the ability to do things that I could never have done by myself.

8.6 Detachment

I have had to detach from some people in my life after coming into recovery. There are people who are just not good for me to be around. I don't think that I could be drawn back into drinking if I was with them but a lot of those friendships were based on drinking. Now that I have put the drink down, we don't have so much in common.

Our fellowship was based around drinking and bars so without that common interest, it is difficult for me to relate as we once did. I have had to detach and keep my distance even though I still think about them, care about them and would like to continue the friendships.

The best way I can love them is to stay sober and stay out of their lives unless one of them reaches out to me for help with their addiction.

In my drinking, I easily became attached to the wrong people so now I seek to associate myself to people who are on the same path of recovery. Rather than drag me down these friends pull me up and support me in my recovery and although I miss the barroom banter, I know that detachment is the safest option for me.

8.7 Emotional Hangovers

Since I got sober, I have not had one single hangover. No more lost days trying to make it through the day on painkillers and antacids. However, what I do still get are emotional hangovers as a result of high doses of negative emotions. Feelings of fear, anxiety, worry, stress and anger all have a way of leaving me tired and washed out.

I can't always avoid these stressful feelings as they are part of life but what I can do is to recognise their effects and look after myself as I recover. When I am emotionally hungover, I need to rest, relax and let go.

I find that anger is particularly exhausting and draining so I need to be very careful with it. Basically, anger and resentment are luxuries that I can't afford as a recovering alcoholic. They are so emotionally draining and too expensive for me in terms of the cost to my peace and sense of well-being.

My emotional hangovers have physical consequences such as headaches and fatigue as well as low mood, so I have to be careful. Of course, they are minor compared with the physical damage and punishment inflicted by alcohol in its hangovers.

I still have days where I marvel at being able to wake up with a clear head and a clear conscience as I am no longer living with the effects of alcoholic drinking. The occasional emotional hangover is a small price to pay in sobriety.

8.8 Maximum Insecurity

One of the effects of my drinking was that I was able to create a feeling of maximum insecurity in those around me. Drinking could make me unpredictable and this produced an underlying and perhaps subconscious sense of insecurity in my family.

Even I didn't know how I was going to be when I was under the influence of alcohol. Generally, I just loved everybody although very occasionally it could make me difficult and awkward. With alcohol in the driving seat, I thought I was okay and that I could handle it but I could not fully trust myself if I was taking alcohol on board.

Sober I am reliable, trustworthy and as honest as anyone else but my drinking eroded my dependability and I think that over time this made for maximum insecurity in myself and in those around me.

Nowadays with a good bit of recovery under my belt, I feel like I am a much safer person and I don't think that I am spreading the underlying feelings of insecurity to my family as I was before.

I feel much more solid, dependable and reliable than I have ever been.

8.9 Intimacy

Drinking cut me off from people especially those I love and those who love me. I knew that when I took a drink, I was separating myself and setting myself apart in all my relationships. There was a physical and spiritual separation taking place that was very destructive to any form of real intimacy.

Physically I needed to separate so that I could drink the way that I wanted to and I practised social distancing because my breath was so heavily laced with alcohol. Spiritually, I knew that I was cutting myself off from God and the more I drank the more distant he became.

At one point I almost lost my faith altogether and I started to wonder if I had just been deluded about faith and God. If there was a God, why had he allowed me to get into this mess and why hadn't he got me out of it?

I am slowly learning to be more intimate in my relationships and I am less distant than I used to be. I also feel less lonely and more connected to other people than before. I am now able to feel and receive love.

Importantly my connection and intimacy with God has been restored and this is so important to me now. I don't want to cut myself off from God or other people anymore and I don't have to as long as I don't take a drink.

8.10 Great Expectations

At school, I had to read the book Great Expectations by Charles Dickens. Being dyslexic, I didn't get much beyond the front cover, but that cover was important because the title has stayed with me.

I have always had such great expectations of life, of others, and of myself. The problem has been that they have often been unrealistic expectations and they have led to a lot of disappointment and discouragement, as well as more drinking. I have heard drinking described as a disease of more, and that rings true for me when I think of the former hopes and dreams that I had for my life.

I could never be content with what I had and I realise that I was always demanding more out of life and out of myself. I still have great expectations but now I seek to direct most of my hopes for the future in the spiritual rather than the material realms of life.

Today I am seeking more peace and a bigger heart of love for those around me.

8.11 The Obsession to Drink

The obsession to drink is one of the chief characteristics of alcoholism. Listening to other people's stories has helped me to see that although it manifests in different ways it is the common denominator in all true alcoholics. For me, it was the ever-present persistent thought about when I could get a drink? Not just a few drinks but saturation drinking up to the level that I wanted.

To do the job properly I needed to be on my own or with other serious drinkers so that I could drink the way I wanted without other people's judgement or censure. For me, the obsession was like a toothache that was always there in the background with daily pain levels fluctuating in intensity between extreme and moderate.

I don't think I realised how powerful the obsession was until I stopped drinking. It was only then that I realised how much drinking alcohol had governed my thinking and my being. It was like a controlling spirit that was always there in the background flexing its muscles, waiting for the starting pistol, pressing and pushing its predictable agenda.

Alcohol was bullying me, enforcing its rule, assuming the right to dominate my being, controlling me and driving my obsession to drink.

8.12 A Change of Perspective

In alcoholism, I was looking through life's binoculars the wrong way and everything was limited and small. But when I stopped drinking, I turned them around and everything looked brighter, clearer and more interesting. I stopped looking through the alcoholic lens of gloom, doom and negativity where I was always thinking that things were getting worse and never better. The glass was always half empty never half full.

Alcohol distorted my whole perspective on life to such an extent that I always assumed that life was getting worse and continually going downhill. I looked back with nostalgia to the good old days but could not look to the present and tomorrow with a positive perspective.

When I was drinking it was almost impossible to look forward with hope and the positive expectation that things were going to improve and get better. It was also totally impossible to comprehend the idea that I could genuinely improve. The song 'things can only get better' used to bug me as it didn't seem to be working out for me. I had found God but I couldn't shake off the ball and chain of my alcoholism. It would always drag me down and cast shadows over my vision of the future.

There have been setbacks in my recovery and there are days when I am looking at life through the wrong lens, but the overall trend is upwards. Year on year life is getting better and I am invested in the future. I no longer live in the past and I am seeking to embrace the changes that life brings.

I am learning to rejoice in the new day and the new opportunities it brings for growth and positive change. I am changing and being changed for the better through the circumstances of my life.

They are working for my good, for my upgrade and preparing me for a heather life that is yet to come.

8.13 Alcoholic Head

Waking up worried and in a negative frame of mind was normal for me. Some days I would wake up with an overwhelming sense of despair and hopelessness. Feeling afraid of the future, aware of the shortness and futility of life, seeing only the things that could go wrong and with darkness closing in. At such times the shadow of death and decay was upon me. This was my alcoholic head. It is no wonder that I used to make straight for the bottle and the escape hatch at every possible opportunity.

Having listened to the stories of many other alcoholic sufferers this appears to be a common symptom. It requires a definite program of action to counter it because even now in recovery listening to my alcoholic head is not a good idea. I have to break out of the negative bubble and this involves disciplines like reading, meditation and prayer. My alcoholic mind needs daily medication and treatment if it is not to take me off down some negative pathway of catastrophe thinking.

This innate negativity needs challenging and I have to ask it some subversive questions. Does this hopeless scenario that I have painted in my mind have to be the potential outcome? Will the future really be worse all the time? Could the future be better rather than worse? My stinking thinking has to be challenged and replaced or it will bring me down.

My alcoholism is not just a physical ailment, it is a deeply rooted mental and spiritual disease that requires a daily program of treatment. Projecting the worst and expecting things to go wrong or to fail, is not the way forward for my alcoholic head. Nowadays, I am giving myself permission to believe that my journey in life can be a happy and joyous one if I go the right way. If I follow the signposts and no longer deliberately ignore them. If I go the way that I am being directed, then I know that my alcoholic head is no longer running the show and I am in a good position to find the life that I am meant to have.

A life filled with joy, freedom and happiness instead of misery, anxiety and pain.

8.14 On My Knees

I have always resisted getting down on my knees to pray and I could give you all sorts of reasons why I don't think it is necessary. However, I have decided to set aside all my clever talk and get down on my knees every day to ask God to help me.

Why the change? The answer is that I was in a recovery meeting and someone who was a newcomer shared that they didn't really have any idea who God is, but in desperation, he decided to get down on his knees every morning and to ask God to help him. Five weeks later and his life was transformed from total carnage to the recovery of his job, his family and his life.

I was really impressed by his utter conviction and his humility to get down on his knees and pray. I thought that if he can do it, and if it worked for him, why don't I just try it? What have I got to lose? I didn't do it immediately but a few weeks later while I was on holiday, I was thinking about it. I was thinking about the things in front of me especially difficult decisions at work and I was feeling out of my depth. I realised that I can't do it on my own. I need a higher power and for me that power is God. I decided that when I got home, I would get down on my knees every morning and ask God to show me the way through the day and to give me the wisdom and guidance that I needed.

I have common sense and I can reason things out, but so many things in life are way beyond my power. My work is in many ways impossible and I need Gods help and guidance in all that I turn my hand to. Getting on my knees is a sign that I am serious about doing business with God and doing God's business.

On my knees, I am humbling my heart, my mind and my body before him and acknowledging that he is God and that I am not. As I arise from my knees, I am excited to see what he is going to do today in my life and in the lives of those around me.

8.15 Imaginary Difficulties

When things are going well and I have no particular immediate problems to handle I find myself getting uneasy. I start to imagine future scenarios where I will not be able to cope. I start to plan and scheme about how I am going to prepare for this imaginary difficulty that I have just created.

In this way, I continually sabotage the present by projecting into an imaginary future. It needs to be said that this imaginary future is always full of disaster and difficulty. In it, I am inevitably struggling to cope and therefore I must prepare myself now. This means that I start clearing the decks so that I can be ready for the imaginary problem when it hits. I will do next week's work now so that I will have time to field the imaginary problem that must surely take place.

I can't enjoy the present moment and the peace that it brings because my mind is now firmly focused on the imaginary future. This is of course all a ridiculous waste of time but it's what I do. I also suspect it's what many others do, particularly people like myself who are caught up in addictive patterns of thought.

This is overthinking on steroids and as with steroids, long-term use causes damage. It puts me under self-imposed stress and I have paid the price which in my own case was in the form of a minor stroke. Much of the stress was self-generated and even the parts that were real, I experienced more intensely than was good for me.

I have had to learn to deal with this dysfunctional thinking as I can no longer take a drink to shut it all off. I now seek to keep life in the day and discipline myself when I find that I am projecting imaginary future life events.

This is all part of my recovery from alcoholism and alcoholic thinking which is rightly called stinking thinking.

8.16 My Place

I have learned to know and value my place in life and I no longer try to run away from where I am meant to be. Sometimes I think that maybe I could get a cottage and hideaway in the countryside or the seaside for the rest of my life. Perhaps I could run away from life's difficulties and just hide?

I suppose that is what I was doing with drink, just hiding from the world and retreating into an altered state of consciousness where I could find some shelter from the realities of life.

Now I live in the real world and I know that escape to the countryside or the bottle will not change things. I will still be there and the answer is to change myself and then to use my place to its maximum advantage.

Even the difficult things and the challenges of my place in life are here to help me to grow and develop. They are as a friend of mine calls them my 'grace growers. People, places and things that stand in front of me and challenge me are there to grow me in grace.

Everything works together for good if I am willing to stick with it and work through things rather than running away.

I no longer desire to run away because I know that deep down this is my place until my higher power calls time and moves me on. I don't have to worry about it as he has the map and compass, not me.

Knowing that I am in the right place, that my life is exactly how it is meant to be and that I have permission to enjoy it is one of the great treasures of my recovery.

8.17 Nothing is Wasted

Nothing is wasted in the economy of God. Even our mistakes, losses and failures can be used by God in the most remarkable ways. Falls from grace accompanied by apparent or real failure can form part of our treasure chest of experience that can be brought out and used to help others at just the right time.

One of the people whose moral failure helped me was Charles Colson, who had been President Nixon's lawyer and right-hand man. He had been convicted of perjury as part of the Watergate scandal and ended up being jailed and stripped of everything. His apparent fall became the source of his life's work as he began to work at every level for prisoners and prison reform in the United States and all around the world.

When I heard him speak, he had just been to Northern Ireland and was working for peace and reconciliation amongst the hunger strikers in the H Block prisons of Northern Ireland. I remember he said that nobody's life is wasted when it is given to God, and that struck a chord with me. It was a significant statement that has been part of me ever since.

I didn't go to jail but I did fall into the prison of alcoholism. I haven't been able to make any difference to the plight of alcoholics at a national or international level but my experience has been of use locally. Even my most difficult experiences of struggle with this disease have not been wasted. Just about every negative experience of my years as an alcoholic drinker have been turned around and used for good.

Nothing is wasted with God, everything is used.

8.18 Bottled Up

Growing up in a household where anger was expressed physically, vocally, violently, explosively and unpredictably, I did not want anger to be part of my life. My mother said that she had grown up in a house where there was never even a raised voice and that became my goal, I wanted to live in peace with those around me.

What I now realise is that I didn't eradicate my anger, I just suppressed it and bottled it up, so it had to find other outlets. Instead of learning healthy ways to acknowledge and express my anger, it turned inwards so that I would focus on beating myself up rather than expressing my anger and then directing it towards a legitimate target.

I drank on my anger and resentments rather than learning how to process them and deal with them in an appropriate manner. But of course, drinking only relieved the pressure temporarily and my anger and resentments would build to explosive levels. The pressure had to find a way out and if it wasn't released through getting drunk, I would get irritable and sensitive to the slightest criticism. Stuffing my anger inside and bottling it up in this way was not healthy and when I came into recovery, I began to recognise my anger and even express it verbally in ways that I had not been able to before.

I remember losing my temper with someone in a public meeting and the strange thing was that it felt good. It was a bit over the top but in my outburst years of pent-up anger and frustration were released. Instead of acting in and taking the anger into myself, I let it out.

It has not been all plain sailing since then but I now recognise my anger and resentments and I seek to deal with them in healthy and appropriate ways. I have to because I am no longer using alcohol to bottle it all up.

8.19 You Haven't Got It

The disease of alcoholism is one that constantly tells you that you haven't got it. It's a fight and a battle that you don't even realise that you are in until you try to stop drinking.

Stopping drinking was never a problem for me until I tried to stop and then I realised that I had a problem. I had been living under the illusion that I could give up any time I wanted but because I didn't want to give up, I hadn't. What I didn't realise was that I couldn't quit because I had a disease that had progressed to a point where it was going to need specialist treatment.

Even when I started to get help and got involved in recovery meetings my mind was constantly arguing with the diagnosis and telling me that I wasn't really an alcoholic and that I was taking all this recovery business too seriously. The disease would be telling me that it really didn't need treatment, that I could happily live with it and that it wasn't necessary for me to take the drastic step of following a total abstinence recovery program.

My alcoholism is still telling me that I am all right and that after all this time it would be quite reasonable for me to take the occasional drink now and then. It tells me that it would be fine to let my hair down occasionally, in fact, it would be quite a good thing to do and that I might find that I was cured and that I can now drink like a normal person.

The longer I go on in sobriety the more I find that alcohol plays this trump card trying to goad me into believing that I haven't got the disease of alcoholism. It wants me to abandon my recovery and to believe the lie that I haven't really got this disease.

Thankfully I know that this is just not true and that I really do have the disease of alcoholism which means that I can never drink again unless I want to risk everything that I have worked for over many years in recovery.

8.20 Thinking Like That

I was having a conversation with someone at the university and she commented to me about something that I had just said, with the words 'I don't think like that'. Nobody had ever said that to me before and it was quite a revelation to meet someone who was thinking about the way they were thinking and was also prepared to challenge me about my way of thinking.

I can't even remember what the subject of the conversation was but that was not the point. The issue was my thinking and she had the courage to challenge me about it by telling me that she didn't think like that. In fact, she had made a decision not to think like that and to think differently.

I was just getting free of my alcoholic drinking at the time and it was an important comment because I began to see just how defective much of my thinking was. In the rooms of recovery, they call it 'stinking thinking' and I was about to be baptised into a wealth of unwanted enlightenment about my distorted patterns of thinking.

Until I entered into recovery I had not been in an environment where my thinking about myself and my life had been deeply questioned. Recovery involves honesty and it wasn't long before people began to challenge my thinking even without them knowing that they were doing so.

I had taken over as literature secretary of a group and I was so proud of myself for having sorted out the books and all the old debris in the suitcase in which they were kept. I told the previous literature secretary what I had done and I suppose that I was quietly boasting about the improvements that I had made. I was expecting and waiting for a load of compliments and praise for my brilliance. Instead, she just looked at me and said 'what do want a medal?' It was a big dose of truth as I realised that in my thinking I was looking for and wanting to be praised and appreciated for just doing my job.

I began to see how in lots of other areas I was requiring and even demanding praise and thanks for doing things that I should have been doing anyway. This was just the beginning of the opening up of new ways of seeing and thinking that are part and parcel of my recovery.

8.21 Wrestling with the Program

A program is a series of steps that can be taken to deal with a problem or produce the desired result. The program of recovery that I follow is the 12-step recovery program developed by Alcoholics Anonymous. I have been in this program for many years now and it has enabled me to stay free of alcohol as well as helping me to deal with the underlying roots of my alcoholism.

The thing about the program that is difficult to understand is that it only continues to work if I work it. The minute I let up on it my recovery starts to slip even if I don't realise it. Very subtly the obsession and the compulsion that drove my drinking starts to return. Initially, it manifests in other obsessive and compulsive behaviours like buying things or exercising obsessively. These for me are warning signs that I have been letting up on my program, usually because I have let it slip from first place in my life.

A sort of fatigue can set in and the meetings that were so exciting and life-giving become boring and tedious. The initial thrill of recovery wears off and the foundational habits of recovery start to slip.

After about seven years in recovery, I pretty much dropped out of the program. I wasn't drinking, life was full and busy and I was involved in helping other alcoholics on a more professional basis. I thought to myself, do I still have to do this? So, I decided to do recovery my way until I hit a crisis point after about eighteen months.

I had been transferring my obsessive and compulsive desire to my religious work but a family crisis tipped me over into a chasm of anxiety and fear from which I couldn't escape. I realised that I needed to return to the program and make it central to my life if I was going to avoid falling back into addiction.

I realised the truth of what I had been told which is that we are not cured of alcoholism, we are just given a daily reprieve conditional on following the steps of the program. The program deals with the roots not just the symptoms.

Dealing with the symptoms without a program is like trying to push a load of floating plastic ducks underwater. You just manage to get two or three down and another one pops up and escapes. Push down one addiction and another one pops up.

Most people wrestle with the program and argue with it at various points in their recovery, but I am now convinced that the power of the program and the power of God that is behind it is essential for the ongoing maintenance of my recovery from addiction and alcoholism.

8.22 Self-Destructive Thinking

Harsh criticism was the backdrop to my life as a child and growing up in such a critical environment made me highly sensitive to criticism. This family culture of intense criticism has been a very destructive force in my life because not only has it deposited within me an overly critical outlook towards others, it has also made me excessively self-critical and harsh on myself.

My constantly running mental tape tends to be negative and highly self-critical as I repeatedly engage in a form of mental self-destruction. I am excessively critical of myself and I am hard-wired to think negatively about who I am and what I do.

In recovery, I have been alerted to these destructive ways of thinking and I now take intentional steps in the opposite direction. At the end of each day, as I review all that has taken place, I purposely bring to mind things that I have done where I can allow myself to feel good about myself. As I focus on these things, I find that my thinking and corresponding feelings start to shift away from the highly critical and self-destructive groove that I have been schooled in and locked into.

The other side-effect of this practice is that I am much less critical and judgemental of others, both in the family and at work. I have also found myself living for and promoting a less critical and judgemental culture in my home life and my workplace.

By tackling my negative and self-destructive thinking I know that I am undermining and disempowering my self-destructive alcoholic mindset and this keeps me one step further away from a drink.

8.23 Holy Communion

As a priest, my job requires me to celebrate Holy Communion, the Eucharist or the Mass as it is called in Roman Catholic circles. This has been really problematic as my job requires me to eat the bread and drink the wine before distributing it to the congregation. Most of the time I have just pretended to drink the wine by putting the cup to my lips and at other times I have let the tiniest quantity of wine rest on my tongue before taking the bread.

Over the last few years, I have not taken the wine at all. A global pandemic meant that as priests we were forbidden to distribute the wine to the congregation at communion and so the problem was pretty much solved for me at a practical level.

Theologically it has been more tricky because I am supposed to be partaking in the blood of Christ and as the president, I am to participate fully in the communion and also but to be the first one to do so. As an alcoholic priest, it is a real dilemma and there is no easy answer.

The deciding factor for me was early one Sunday morning when I was celebrating Holy Communion alone because no one else had turned up at church and I was really tempted to down the whole cup. I took the wine before the wafer and as I did so a trickle went down the back of my throat. I felt the burn. What a way to be tempted in the most sacred of situations possible? It freaked me out as I realised then that I was playing with fire and that I needed to review my practice.

At the same time, I also heard a recovery speaker share their experience of this and their decision not to take the wine, even to their lips or onto their tongue. This convinced me that for my own safety I would only take communion in one kind in the form of the bread.

Some people use non-alcoholic wine but that presents all sorts of problems in a small congregation and the non-alcoholics like their slug of full-strength communion wine. So, I just don't take the communion wine which is a decision that I am at peace with as it is the safest option.

8.24 Making Nothing Happen

I wanted to be a successful priest and I wanted my Church to be a successful church. By successful, I mean a lively community of faith with lots of people as well as being the sort of church that people really want to belong to. With the best of intentions both myself and the team working alongside me ended up pushing, forcing and imposing our wills on the situation. We were trying to make something happen by using our own abilities and gifts and despite some initial apparent success it just wasn't working.

The fallout was painful and very costly in terms of personal relationships, reputations and finances. When I was in the depth of despair about the situation, I was given a book by a colleague of mine which had the title 'making nothing happen.' The content of the book was unimportant but the title began to speak to me as it jutted out from my bookshelf. I realised that we had been imposing our will on the situation by trying to make something happen and it hadn't worked, in fact, it had been blocked.

As I reflected on this and the book title, I realised that I had not been going about this the right way. I had been bombarding the situation with willpower, by trying to make something happen when it clearly wasn't. All it did was produce trouble and conflict instead of peace and healthy growth.

The idea of making nothing happen was pretty alien to me but the title started to get into my bones as I realised that instead of making room for God, I had filled up the creative space with a program that was actually blocking the flow of Gods grace. It was like trying to cut against the grain and I had to learn to go with the grain.

What I learned through this is to have the courage of my convictions and to go with God even if that means making nothing happen.

8.25 Running and Drinking

For many years I used running as a way of reigning in my addiction to alcohol. Running was a way for me to put my compulsive and obsessive energies to use in a more positive and healthy way.

When I was marathon training, I would run for up to four hours at a time until I was so exhausted that all I could do afterwards was to eat and sleep. It was a way to avoid drinking as it provided an all-consuming substitute activity that seemed to do the job, at least for a while.

I have met a number of people who run drug and alcohol addiction recovery programs that are based on running as a substitute for drinking and using. The running also releases endorphins which give the runners high where you can feel elated and have a greatly heightened mood as a consequence of such a large or intense dose of exercise.

Of course, running didn't stop me from drinking it just helped me to put the brakes on it. It also offered a temporary release from the pressure to drink although my attendance at the local running club undid a lot of this positive benefit as training sessions would invariably end up in the bar.

One of the unforeseen consequences of this running is that it provided a smokescreen for my drinking because it was difficult to imagine how someone could be such a keen runner and an alcoholic at the same time.

As I look back, I can see that I was cross-addicted as I had transferred my addiction to alcohol over to physical exercise addiction. I approached running in the same way that I approached drinking. It was an all or nothing business with no half measures. Within a short time of starting out with the running club, I was already aiming at marathon distances as a meagre five-kilometre race was just not enough.

The running also provided a way of clearing my head after a heavy evening of drinking so that I could think more clearly. I have met quite a few alcoholics who have used running as a way of trying to control their drinking but in the end, most of them have had to quit running due to overuse injuries or age.

One of my running buddies used to say that if you run you can eat and drink what you like. It didn't work out that way for him as he ate and drank what he liked then had a heart attack and died too soon.

8.26 See Me

Before I came into recovery a good friend of mine who has known me since I was a teenager said to me 'Chris, you are trying to be something that you are not.' This comment really struck home because I felt that there was truth in it. I was finding it difficult to be myself and to be honest in expressing who I really was to the people around me.

I felt that if I told them who I really was then that would not be good enough for them because I would not be who they wanted me to be. I did not feel safe to let on who I was or what I really thought, so there was fundamental dishonesty at work in all my relationships. This dishonesty and pretence meant that I would do things or behave in ways that would be seeking to gain the approval of others, but in the process, I was crushing and denying my true self. In fact, I ended up not really knowing who I was or what I was doing as I desperately sought to be who you wanted me to be and to do what you wanted me to do.

All the time I was trying to hide and cover up my alcoholism, I was presenting a false self in order to stop you from seeing the real me. I was afraid that you might see me and that if you saw the real me you would reject me and I would fail to gain your acceptance and approval which I desperately needed. My need for your acceptance and approval was so strong and it would constantly lead me into compromise and situations where people would manipulate me because of my need for their approval.

Now I have been honest about alcohol I am gaining the courage, to be honest about many other things. I am increasingly coming from a place of true honesty and reality as I am no longer trying to be something that I am not. I am who I am and if you don't like me then that is your problem, not mine. The best thing that I can do for you is to be true to myself.

8.27 Feeling different

I don't think that alcoholics are alone when they say that for a lot of their lives, they have felt different. I am sure that many people feel different from the people around them at various times in their lives, however, many alcoholics testify to feeling different a lot of the time.

I have experienced this many times throughout my life particularly at school and then at work. Drinking enabled me to feel less different and more in tune with the people around me but when it wore off things just went back to how they were before.

I was aware that I came across as a bit odd to people and I know that this was often the way that I was perceived. I didn't want to be different or to feel different but I couldn't avoid it. I would usually experience life as an outsider rather than an insider and I didn't feel part of any group even when I wanted to.

It wasn't until about nine years into my recovery that this sense of feeling different started to melt in the rooms of recovery. Something changed, maybe it was me, as I began to feel part of rather than an outsider in the rooms. I started to feel that I belonged and was able to receive the love that was being extended to me. I also began to really love and appreciate my fellow travellers in a way that I hadn't before.

It has been a really wonderful experience to feel that I am no longer different and odd. I may still be different but that is not how I am treated or how I feel when I am in my recovery group. As I look around the recovery room, I can see quite a few other people who are different or even odd but I just love being with them because I too am one of them. They are my people, my tribe and like me, many have spent their whole lives feeling different.

It is an amazing thing after all these years as an outsider to be with people who feel the same as I do and who I can feel totally at ease with.

This is one of the miracles of recovery. Being able to belong to a group of people without feeling different.

8.28 A Thankful Heart

One of the significant changes that have taken place in my recovery is a change of heart. I find myself with a heart full of gratitude and spilling over with thanksgiving.

My prayers are often little more than 'thank you, God, thank you, thank you, thank you!'

This is not just a seasonal high but a new disposition that has been deposited in me by God. It is a new heart of gratitude and love for God that I didn't have before. I don't have to manufacture this or work it up because it comes from within as I find this spirit of gratitude and thankfulness just welling up from inside me.

Even if things are not going that well or not going my way it is still there bubbling away in the background. It's a sort of continual but delightful hum in the background that is just audible in my heart. It's such a better spirit than the one that used to rule and dominate my life.

Alcohol is a hard taskmaster and is used to continuously beat me down and keep me low. I would live in a sea of negativity and always see what was missing rather than what I had actually been given.

The wonderful thing about my gratitude is that I don't need external things, situations or substances to make me happy. The happiness is on the inside as my spirit is alive to God. It is like having a permanent celebration, a praise party going on deep down in my heart so that no matter what is going on around me I can still rejoice in my inner being.

I admit that to many people this must sound like crazy stuff but it is my experience and it's wonderful. I want other people to know this for themselves and to know that there is no limit to what is available to us in the world of the spirit.

The resources of God are limitless.

8.29 Not Bad Enough

It was difficult to really join a recovery group because I felt that my drinking was not bad enough for me to qualify as a member. I hadn't been taking cocaine or getting up in the night to drink and I hadn't been arrested or sectioned under the mental health act. I hadn't been homeless or jobless and I hadn't been drinking in the morning before work. I'd also been avoiding driving with a drink inside me and so for all these kinds of reasons I thought that I could not be a member of Alcoholics Anonymous. My drinking just wasn't bad enough for me to qualify for membership.

It was only when I found out that the only qualification for membership was having a desire to stop drinking that I began to wonder if I could join. Again, I wasn't really sure that I qualified because although I wanted to cut down and eliminate some of the more unpleasant consequences like hangovers, I didn't want to stop entirely.

That thinking all changed in the last few months before I came into recovery. During that time, I realised that whilst I sincerely believed I could stop, I could not imagine life without alcohol and without the facility to get drunk as getting drunk had always been my major solution to most of my life's problems. I don't know how it happened but in the last days of my drinking I became confident that I would be able to stop but I was going to need help staying stopped as this was something that I had never managed to achieve.

My drinking was bad enough for me to know that although I could just about stop for a time, I couldn't let it go completely. It had a hold on me so that no matter what I tried I would always return to drinking and end up drunk. Strange as it may seem this was my ticket to Alcoholics Anonymous membership.

This was bad enough to allow me access into this most elite of clubs.

8.30 Alcoholic Excitement

Living in an alcoholic environment with an active alcoholic comes with its own unique level of craziness. With an alcoholic in the house, there is an excitement, a constant sense of drama and the feeling that something is happening or just about to happen. Living with this chaotic buzz of uncertainty and alcoholic energy just becomes so normal that it only becomes really noticeable when the alcoholics' presence is withdrawn.

When my dad used to go away travelling with his work, a sense of peace and tranquillity would descend on our house and we would all relax. I still remember the summer holidays when my dad was away and it was just me, my brother and my mum at home. It was so peaceful, relaxed and laid back.

When my dad came back everything would once again become turbocharged and whilst it was at times exciting, it was like living with a perpetual thunderstorm, complete with torrential rain and wind. It was dramatic and unpredictable but also destabilising. He brought an energy but it was a restless energy that was fuelled by the disease.

It was impossible to relax with my dad in the house as he was so driven and restless. In fact, none of us was allowed to relax when he was around as he had to keep us all busy. Even trying to watch the television together was difficult as it was pre-remotes so we would be constantly ordered to get up and change the channels for him.

I didn't begin to understand all this until years later when I started to find recovery myself. My alcoholism gave me the same sort of restless spirit and one of the consequences of this was that I couldn't sit still. I was constantly fidgeting and tapping or drumming with my fingers.

Even now I'm recovery this restlessness has not entirely gone and I can sometimes find it hard to relax but I no longer transmit that restlessness to those around me. I am calmer, more peaceful and relaxed than I was. I think the keyword is serenity which is one of the most valued fruits of my recovery.

I don't miss the highly charged atmosphere of my alcoholic home and I am slowly learning to relax and make nothing happen even if it can at times seem a little dull in comparison to alcoholic chaos.

8.31 Acquisition of a Higher Power

Instead of a can or a bottle in my hand, I now have a living, breathing, walking, talking moment by moment personal dealing with the unseen God. I now have an effective faith in a power greater than myself. It's a faith that works at the level of ordinary life. I have a power in my life that does for me what I could never do by myself.

Today I have the help and strength of Gods power in my life. It's not just a theory but a reality. I live in the awareness of God's manifest loving presence who is helping me to live well in this world. I am constantly amazed that God is with me in this personal and intimate way.

I don't think that this is an unusual or unique experience as I meet a lot of people in recovery who are on the same sort of journey with God. The God idea really works for me because I am holding onto him in the same way that I used to hold onto the bottle.

Now that I am holding onto God, I am no longer putting my faith in the next drink. I am not relying on alcohol but on God's strength and his courage. Instead of the hiss of the ring pull, I now pray and then drink deeply, gulping down a much better and stronger spirit. I was always thirsty but now I assuage that thirst with a spiritual drink instead of alcohol.

Alcohol was my higher power and I put my faith in bottles and cans but now my faith is in a power that is much stronger than alcohol. Now when I see someone walking around clutching a can of beer and holding onto it for security, I say a prayer for them. I ask my higher power that they too might come to know the liberation and real security that comes from putting our faith in a power greater than ourselves, not alcohol but God.

September

9.1 Relationship or Religion

My religion and my religious devotions did not enable me to break free from alcoholism. You would think that being a priest would put you in a favourable position with God and that he would bring the required release, but this was not how it worked out for me. Although I did find recovery, I didn't find it in the church. I found many good things in church but the connection with God that I was seeking there, mostly eluded me.

In the rooms of recovery, I met people who clearly had a good connection as they spoke of his actions in their daily lives in a way that was rare in my religious tradition. In my religion, we have a lot of theory but these alcoholics spoke of their daily encounters, dealings and direction from a higher power who many, but by no means all, call God.

This was what I had been looking for all along and although I had some experience of it in my religion it was not something that I had been able to hold onto. Strange as it may seem I had to go to the rooms of alcohol recovery to find the relationship with God that I had been looking for all my life. In those rooms, I started to experience a deep sense of Gods peace and rest. Gradually the door opened wider so that I was able to experience more of His presence, not only in the rooms but outside as well.

This was all outside the walls of my religion where there were no priests or theological experts, just fellow travellers who had found a way into a relationship with

God that really worked for them. It worked for me too as I found that in the rooms of Alcoholics Anonymous, I could connect with God in a way that I could not in my religious system, even as a priest.

Today I have a living relationship with God that transcends my religious tradition as I now know the reality of God in the centre of my being in a way that I never did before coming into recovery.

9.2 Caretaking

Coming from an alcoholic family I have an irrational and disproportionate desire to take care of other people's feelings. In the process of caretaking, I have walked all over my own boundaries and failed to look after myself. I have been constantly trying to make everyone else feel good and I have had a desperate desire to keep everybody happy.

Instead of living my own life, I have ended up living theirs as I have been taking care of their feelings and focusing on them. My mindset has been overly responsible for other people's feelings and I have found myself living life to please them instead of living to please God.

Not wanting to upset them or cause ripples in the relationship I have willingly put up with their unacceptable behaviour. I used to think that I would some way be able to control their feelings by my reactions and behaviour.

This illusion of being able to look after or superintend other people's feelings was of course not real. It came from my early home life where I thought that if I behaved exactly as my father wanted then I would be able to control his temper and his behaviour in the home.

I was under the illusion that I could control the atmosphere in the house by my caretaking. I spent my life at home thinking that I was caretaking and managing my father's feelings through my behaviour.

This pattern of caretaking didn't work then and it doesn't work now as I can't control another person's feelings. All it does is make me their slave as I sacrifice my own life in a vain attempt to manage their feelings. I have to avoid offending them or upsetting them and work my whole life around trying to soothe them and make their life better regardless of the cost to me as a person.

The cost of this has been high in terms of resentments as I have stuffed my feelings towards those that I have been trying to caretake. This has all been the fuel to the fire of my drinking. It was only when drinking that I could temporarily detach from this warped way of thinking and living.

I find it all too easy to fall back into caretaking mode when it comes to other people's feelings. The fact is that now I do sometimes have to upset other's feelings as I do what is right for me in any given situation.

9.3 The Damage

In the alcohol Detox Unit where I work as a chaplain, I meet people with liver problems and some of these people have yellow skin. This is the result of jaundice which is a consequence of alcohol or drug-induced liver damage. Cirrhosis of the liver, pancreatitis, hepatitis, ascites, peripheral nerve damage, wet brain, and injuries through seizures and strokes are just some of the consequences of alcohol addiction. These physical consequences are bad enough but there are also rafts of serious mental problems that slowly start to manifest in active addiction. Much of this damage is masked by medication but the damage that alcohol can inflict on the human body and mind is colossal.

Following a stroke, I found myself in a hospital ward with a very young man who was dying of end-stage liver failure brought on by alcohol. He was continuously vomiting and excreting blood and was in intense pain. The liquid morphine that he was being administered by mouth was not even touching his pain. I was there for three days and three nights and I witnessed this young man rapidly deteriorating. His only hope was a liver transplant but because of his history with alcohol, he was not eligible.

His family had gathered around his bed and I was able to give them a glimmer of encouragement but the prognosis was bleak. I prayed a lot for him as I lay in the bed opposite watching him dying in pain. Now whenever I see jaundiced people in the detox centre, I think of him.

That memory spurs me on to help those still suffering from this most relentless of diseases.

9.4 Conscious Contact

I was really surprised in alcohol recovery to find such a strong emphasis on finding and maintaining conscious contact with a higher power. This foregrounding of spirituality was not something that I had expected when I entered the rooms of recovery.

I was amazed at the level of open sharing by members of the group as they talked about the various ways that they had found and were maintaining a living connection with their higher power. I remember sitting there and thinking, if only we could have this kind of honest conversation in the church. As a priest, I have spent hundreds of hours in small talk after church when I have been longing to talk about the things in life and faith that really matter.

People in the rooms weren't talking about the weather because they had something more important to share. It became clear that people in the twelve-step program of recovery were practising prayer and meditation in order to improve their conscious contact with the God of their understanding.

As I attended these meetings it became increasingly apparent that these people were more serious about their spiritual lives than many people in my church. How could this be? The answer was that they had been so desperate that they were willing to give anything a try, even prayer. More than that they were clearly getting results in terms of sobriety and a better way of living than the one they had before.

There was open-mindedness and a spirit of experimentation that was refreshing to me and it opened the door for me to experience a far greater and more consistent conscious contact with God.

I am in no doubt that recovery meetings are a spiritual event and I encounter God in these rooms. It's a spiritual program that works.

9.5 Asking for Help

There came a point in my recovery where I had to ask for and accept help. I could not crack this on my own. Asking for help was not a sign of weakness or failure but an admission of defeat at the hands of a foe who I came to recognise as far more powerful than me.

I don't know why I had not done this before because it was obvious that I could not overcome this affliction on my own. I suppose I was one of those men who would just not go and see the doctor. I thought that I could deal with this by myself and of course, I could not. It's one thing to ask for help but it's another thing altogether to receive the help that is being offered.

Recovery groups deliver what could be called tough love as people get straight to the point. They have to because it is a matter of life and death. We have to tell the truth to one another because the release only comes when we do that. There is no easier or softer way and this is where the concept of sponsorship comes in. This is one member showing another member the way. It is not a set plan or a prescribed route, but a bespoke program individually tailored by God so that we can get the maximum recovery if we want it.

It's not foolproof and some sponsorship arrangements go wrong, but when it works, it is brilliant because it delivers the help that we need, when we need it. My sponsor continues to help me week-by-week as we talk and engage in the conversation of recovery. I am so glad that I had the courage to reach out and ask him for help. It wasn't a sign of weakness but a step of faith that required courage.

I now encourage others who are suffering from this disease not to isolate but to take the free help that is available day and night through twelve-step fellowships.

9.6 No More Hangovers

After a time of not drinking alcohol, it suddenly dawned on me that I had not lost one second of my life to a hangover. No more chronic headaches and dosing up on paracetamol to get through the day. No more night sweats or feeling sick in the morning. No more nights spent with my head down the toilet. What a fantastic release from the alcohol excess of the previous day.

I love going to bed sober and even after all these years in recovery, I still enjoy the novelty of it. I like the fact that my breath never smells of old alcohol and that I am not walking around dehydrated by yesterday's booze. I love being clean and sober.

Interestingly I am still not a morning person but now I sleep properly as there is no alcohol in my system to disrupt my sleep patterns. If I am tired, it's because I have been working not because of staying up late into the night drinking. I am not in the slightest bit worried about getting in the car to drive in the morning. I don't have to build hangover recovery time into my schedule. Not drinking is so freeing and liberating and I love being sober all the time.

Near the end of my drinking, I hated having alcohol in my system, it was like an allergy, but these days I don't have that problem. I can think clearly all the time without the after-effects of alcohol eroding my mental faculties.

Over the last few years, I have hardly ever used headache tablets and I have so much more energy. I love waking up with a crystal-clear head and the complete absence of any sort of hangover. I need never have one again.

9.7 Faith in a Substance

When I was drinking, I was putting my faith in a substance and that substance was alcohol. I was trusting alcohol to do for me what I could not do for myself. I needed alcohol to make me feel normal. I entrusted my emotional life to this substance as I handed over the control of my feelings to it. I could see alcohol and I could feel the effects of alcohol so it seemed real to me and the experiences that it gave me all appeared to be real.

However, alcohol was a liar that masqueraded as my friend and the more I trusted it, the more it was betraying me behind my back. I was putting my faith in the most untrustworthy, unreliable, despicable, and destructive of substances. It seems foolish now and rather obvious that this was a very poor decision, but alcohol is a cunning and deceptive substance that lured me into a false sense of security before turning on me.

I now put all my faith in a higher power and that power is God. Faith is a substance. It's the substance of things hoped for and the promise of things not yet seen. Faith is not such an obvious substance as alcohol but it is just as real.

My faith takes on form and substance as I act on it. The reality of my faith is manifested in my life as I follow its leading and direction. My faith is now real and provides the things that I was looking for in alcohol. My faith and the thinking that is generated from it has the effect of changing the way I feel.

Everything I was looking for alcohol to do for me now comes from a power greater than myself and that power is accessed not by taking a drink but by faith, which when activated becomes substantial.

9.8 Recovering or Recovered

Soon after I started going to recovery meetings, I started to notice that whilst most of the recovering alcoholics described themselves as recovering there was a small minority who used the word recovered. Little did I realise that I had stumbled upon a philosophical division within the recovery community.

Some recovering addicts see themselves as recovered primarily because they are no longer using alcohol or other substances whilst others look on addiction as a lifelong illness for which there is no cure. The latter group would see themselves in remission or as having a reprieve conditional on the maintenance of their program.

I don't know the precise reason why some addicts call themselves recovered or if there is an exact explanation. Perhaps they feel that they have moved on and no longer want to identify with alcohol or drugs as they once used to. However, I think that those of us who have battled this powerful and cunning disease for many years are suspicious about claims that move towards the idea of being cured. We have seen too many people confidently identify as recovered only to fall flat on their faces by going out and getting drunk or worse still staying drunk.

My own personal approach is to say that it is not wise to get into this argument and just to 'live and let live.' Each person can call themselves what they like as long as they can stay sober and not pick up a drink then all is well.

9.9 All the God's

I have heard it said that all the God's send their drunks to Alcoholics Anonymous and I think that there is a good deal of truth in this. My own religion has struggled with the question of what to do with the hopeless alcoholic and I suspect that all the religions struggle with their drunks. Religion feels that it should be able to relieve the alcoholic but as a priest, I know that this is usually not the case.

Alcoholism is no respecter of persons or religions and it is totally indiscriminate when it comes to faith. Faith or no faith alcohol has more than enough power to rule over its unwitting victims. Alcoholics Anonymous is not a religion neither does it promote any particular faith or religious system. The fellowship is comprised of all different religions and denominations and includes many atheists as well as agnostics. It is not gathered around a theology or any particular dogma but is instead formed around a common goal of helping alcoholics to recover from alcoholism.

As a theologian, this is fascinating for me as I hear people from all different faiths and none share about their relationship to a higher power. I regularly have the thought that this shouldn't work but it does, which in my view is a miracle. How can people from all different faiths and belief systems sit in the same room and help each other to get better?

No theological arguments, no preaching, no hierarchy of belief systems, just simple faith in a power great than ourselves who has rescued us from the tyrannical grip of alcoholism. This is the outstanding miracle of Alcoholics Anonymous and one that should make all religious leaders of whatever faith, sit up and take note.

9.10 Those Who Fail

I hate being blamed and I would guess that no one really enjoys taking the blame for anything. Some people are brought up in family cultures where those who fail are not considered worthy of love and they find themselves being blamed and condemned.

We alcoholics can face a lot of blame and condemnation as love is withdrawn or withheld by those close to us who try to control our drinking using the power tools at their disposal. The withdrawal of love and affection by those closest to us is a bitter thing.

We are those who fail and have failed, so we find ourselves condemned and cast out. We become persona non grata as we are cast outside the camp, unclean and rejected like the lepers of old. But with us, there is no sympathy as alcoholism is not seen as a disease but as a self-inflicted injury that we have brought upon ourselves. We are unworthy of love and we are condemned.

Just spend some time in a hospital ward that is being forced to detox a patient and you will know what it is like to be looked down on, to be blamed and condemned. It is not a great experience to be perceived as a total and utter failure.

There are people and places who suspend judgement, who believe in us, and who love us to life. There are people out there who don't blame alcoholics for their disease or condemn us as failures. They believe in us and are prepared to work with us for our recovery.

Thank God for all the people who give their lives to helping us and supporting us through the many ups and downs of alcohol recovery.

9.11 Identifying Myself as an Alcoholic

One of the initial and rather strange experiences of attending local recovery meetings was the ritual of introducing ourselves at the beginning of meetings. This didn't happen in the London meetings that I attended and you would only have to identify as an alcoholic in order to speak.

However, at the local meetings, they would go round the room and I would have to say 'I'm Chris and I'm an alcoholic.' I found it to be a very strange experience, sitting in those rooms and saying those words.

At first, I didn't really want to say them and I found myself saying to myself things like, am I really an alcoholic? Could it be that I am taking all this too seriously? Maybe I should just cool it a bit and let these people do their own thing? Surely, I can't be one of these people?

Interestingly nobody questions you about this or asks for your credentials. It's all about self-identification which happens as you listen to other people's stories. This happened to me big time on my first visit to the rooms. A man shared his story and it was my story, indeed his name was even the same as mine. I knew when I heard him share that I was in the right place. Even though I was reluctant to say it I knew at that moment that this was where I belonged and however strange it might seem I too was an alcoholic.

My reluctance to identify as an alcoholic was not unfounded, as in our society the image of the alcoholic is not a great one and certainly not something you want to put on your job application for being someone's parish priest.

Over time the process of listening to people who have the same kind of characteristics and experience around alcohol was such a relief, as I realised that I wasn't the only one and it explained much of my experience in life so far.

9.12 Superficial Solutions

Recovery from alcoholism is not the result of superficial change as it involves a deep work within us. In order to administer the cure, I had to come to terms with the severity of the disease. I had to accept that my alcoholism is a serious illness that if left untreated will lead to insanity and death. This might seem overdramatic to the outside observer but I know just how deeply rooted this disease is.

For years I fooled myself into thinking that I wasn't too bad and that there were many other people who were worse than me. I thought I would be able to get by and muddle through if I didn't go overboard with my drinking. What I didn't bargain for was that when drinking I had a maniac on board who was hell-bent on destroying everything good in my life. Alcohol was the fifth column constantly betraying me on the inside.

Superficial and external solutions never worked in the long term. The only thing that has worked is continual attention that focuses on the root of the problem. It has of course involved a radical separation from alcohol as a substance and this is something that I was highly resistant to. My alcoholism put up a big fight at the thought of having its power source cut off.

The driving force of alcohol has been stopped as long as I do the work. I need to keep the sea wall in good shape because the tide and the storms are always seeking to erode and undermine my defences against the first drink. My recovery is not a superficial thing, it involves a continuous process of deep inner work and a constant willingness to change.

9.13 The Lifeboat

I love watching lifeboat and helicopter rescue programs on television. I was watching a program featuring a couple of boys who had been stranded on the end of a pier and were clinging on as the tide was sweeping in. Another minute and they would have been swept away to their deaths. They had no idea about how much danger they were in. They had just gone out for a walk on the beach on a sunny day.

This was like me with alcohol, I had no idea of the true nature of the danger that I was in. My whole life was about to be swept away by the riptide of alcoholism. The lifeboat came along just in time for me and I was desperate enough to get on board. I realised that I was in trouble and that I needed to climb aboard. The lifeboat took me to the shore and to dry land. I have found stability and security as I have stayed on the dry land and not ventured out into the seas of drinking once again. I have been miraculously rescued once so I don't want to tempt fate and go back out there again.

Having been rescued in this way it is only natural that I should want to join the lifeboat crew so that I can help to rescue others. What a joy to see someone new climb aboard the lifeboat of recovery and start heading for the shore. There is nothing to beat seeing the gratitude and relief in those who have been rescued from the fierce tides of alcoholism.

9.14 Against the Grain

When I was drinking, I had a sense that I was going against the grain. Rather than going with God, I was refusing to conform to his will for my life. The first step in my new journey with God involved agreeing with him about my drinking. It took me a lifetime of arguing with Him about this before I got into line and decided to go with the grain.

As with wood cutting, going with the grain is a lot easier and more efficient. There is less wasted energy and now when I do swing the axe it seems to be more effective. Life works as it is meant to these days now that I am going with the grain.

I am not battling against the wind of God's will as I used to be in the past. God didn't let me get away with doing life my way. He wanted me to live for him and to do life his way. He stood in my way and blocked me for over fifty years until I finally surrendered to his will for my life.

It is not only in drinking that I was going against the grain but in many other things as well. As I go on in recovery, I increasingly find myself saying 'thy will not my will be done.' Life feels a lot less hard work than it used to and I am finding solutions to my problems in ways that I never used to.

It seems that I am caught up in the flow of Gods Spirit in a way that I was not before. All this has come from a simple willingness to stop resisting and to say yes to God.

9.15 The Pupil is Ready

I've heard it said that when the pupil is ready the teacher will come. It's talking about coming to a place in our lives where we are teachable. It was difficult for God to instruct this know-it-all and therefore he has had to be incredibly patient.

I have had to learn the meaning of this phrase the hard way particularly with respect to alcohol. I just could not be told and was resistant to any idea that it could be bad for me. I was tenacious in my desire to hold onto my drinking come hell or high water.

I remember having to attend a seminar given by a representative of an alcohol and drug rehab. I had been to the pub for a beer before the meeting and dismissed what he said as ridiculous. The pupil was clearly not ready and I had to go out and do more research for myself.

That research involved getting into even greater difficulty with alcohol until I finally had to admit that I had been wrong. I was wrong about alcohol and when I made that admission, I suddenly became teachable. I was no longer sticking my fingers in my ears and I was willing to listen to another point of view.

The teacher came to me in different ways and from different directions. People, books, meetings and just the still small voice deep within. The voice of God that I had drowned out with booze.

When I was ready the teacher came but it had taken most of my life to get to the point where I was truly teachable.

9.16 Respectable People

When I was thinking about what I should be doing as a priest I read some words of Jesus that just leapt out at me. He said 'I have not come to call respectable people but outcasts.' As I read these words, they really impacted me and I sensed that they had my name on them.

I remember wondering what this might mean and why God seemed to be highlighting them. It was especially strange because I was working among highly respectable people who didn't seem to have many problems and they certainly were not outcasts in any shape or form.

From that time onwards God started bringing outcasts to me. They came one by one either to the church building or my house. A young woman who had just broken out of life-long heroin addiction started coming to church. I considered it a great honour that God had sent her to our church and that he trusted us with her. One Sunday morning, I introduced her to a visiting Bishop. I'm not sure what he made of her as she was swaying and slurring her speech being strung out on a high dose of methadone at the time.

God has brought us more than a few alcoholics and quite a few others who did not fit the respectability criteria of the Church of England. In spite of my calling, I'm not saying that I was able to help them all. One of these precious people died of alcohol withdrawal seizures and another died of alcohol-induced cancer.

Even today one of them wanders around my parish as a destitute, living rough in the woods in all weathers. He comes to see me for a chat, usually when he is drunk. He stands right up close and preaches to me from the Bible.

I long for him to find recovery however the reality seems to be that he is getting more and more unwell.

9.17 Pressing On

For years I just kept pressing on with life by moving forward and refusing to look back. In some ways, this wasn't bad as it enabled me to keep going and I was not too bogged down by thinking about the past.

Now as I think about this, I realise that it was ridiculous to think that I could just keep pressing on without addressing my past, especially my alcoholic past. I think that my understanding or should I say misunderstanding of religious conversion had a lot to do with this. I thought that because my past sins were all forgiven, I could just bag up my past, put it in the sin bin and move on. I had no idea that the mess of the early years of my life before my epiphany would need to be worked through and properly put to bed. I had done quite a bit of work on my past with my counsellor before I came into recovery but I never felt that there had been full and final closure following the many hours of talking.

It wasn't until I got a sponsor who took me through the steps that I started the process of working through my past and putting it properly to bed. It took me the best part of a year working with my sponsor to get things straight and to move on. Meeting by meeting we worked through my 'searching moral inventory' as it is called looking at every stage of my life even from before my birth. I was rigorously honest and no stone was left unturned in the process. Every twist and turn of my character found itself being exposed to the light and it was pretty painful at times. None of us likes admitting all our faults and failures, especially to another human being.

When completed it was a liberating experience as I had no more secrets or shame to hide. I had shared my complete truth with another human being and everything was out in the open.

It was a total and complete confession and it liberated me from my bondage to the past.

9.18 Patterns

The advantage of working with my sponsor has been that he really knows me and that means he has been able to help me to live out my recovery. One of the most helpful things that he has been able to do is to point out my defective patterns of thinking and ways of seeing. A good example of this is in the area of self-esteem.

The review of my early life showed how my self-esteem had been smashed to pieces by my father's impossible demands as well as the negative effects of dyslexia in the education system. These two experiences had set me up for a lifetime of warped thinking about myself and my abilities.

The effect of this had been manifested in a continual lack of an appropriate level of self-confidence and as a consequence, I just didn't think I was up to doing life. I also didn't see myself as good enough and therefore I avoided taking responsibility and making decisions. I always deferred to others because I didn't think that I was good enough even though I was usually more than able to do whatever I was being asked to do.

I came to see how this had often frustrated the people around me who wanted me to step up to do things that I was clearly able to do. They would perceive this as a lack of courage but what they didn't see were the inner brakes that were firmly locked on as a result of my childhood.

It took me a long time to absorb what my sponsor was telling me about myself. I just couldn't see what he could see but gradually the light began to dawn and I started to understand and see these patterns for myself.

This has been the deep place of recovery, within me, because this is where the change happens and this is the place of true healing as I have walked out of my previous negative programming to live as a free man.

Recovery doesn't remove my alcoholism but it does reduce the power of my past programming to drive my present life forward in the wrong way.

9.19 Recovery First

As the days become years in recovery, I have to remember that without my sobriety everything is lost. My whole world is now built on the foundations of a non-drinking life, so keeping them well maintained is a priority. This means putting recovery first in my life, and of course, this is a challenge as life takes off and gets busy.

I was recently asked if I would like to consider applying for a new job and it was a very good one. As I reflected on it, I began to see that if I took the job there would have been very little if any time or energy left over for my recovery meetings and commitments. This could have ended up compromising or even jeopardising my ongoing recovery.

The job would have involved working full-time with addicts and people with mental health problems and I realised that for me it was a bridge too far. I would have been too deeply immersed in the world of detoxification, rehabilitation and mental health.

It's tempting to want to dive in and to try to rescue everyone but I need to recognise and know my limits. It's about having the common sense to realise when I am overreaching myself and putting my recovery in danger.

In a way, I do have to accept that I live with limits like anyone with an incurable disease. Most of the time it doesn't affect me but I have to remember to make my recovery a priority and to put my recovery first.

9.20 Different Shapes of Recovery

There is no perfect path to recovery from alcoholism. Some people seem to get it straight away but for most of us, it's a journey that involves both progress and regression. Amongst my friends in recovery, there are life-long slippers alongside people with fifty years of continuous sobriety.

I don't judge anybody else's recovery because I have not walked in their shoes. I don't know what sort of life experience they have had or what difficulties they are seeking to overcome in their lives. We are not all born equal and some people start pretty far back as they are born into dysfunctional families and social worlds that are deeply corrupted.

Some have been trafficked for sex as children, others have grown up with drug-addicted parents and lived chaotic lives. Some have experienced serious mental illness only to be sent out into the community to survive the best they can.

I have great respect for my friends who just can't seem to get continuous sobriety. No matter how much they try permanent abstinence seems to elude them as they fall once again before the power of the bottle.

There are recoveries that go well for many years perhaps twenty-five or thirty years but then for no apparent reason, the person picks up a drink. This is the insanity of the disease of alcoholism as it eludes all rational explanations.

It has many shapes and forms which is why I need to belong to a fellowship that can help to protect me from its chameleon-like and deceptive ways.

9.21 Seeking the Praise

There are dangers in being the leader of anything which is why recovery groups operate a system of rotational leadership so that no one person gets to be put on a pedestal or is allowed to become a dictator.

Service positions in recovery groups have given me the opportunity to develop my skills and abilities in new ways and in a different context. I have found leadership roles in the recovery community to be a lot more straightforward than leadership in a faith community.

This is not to say that service in a recovery group is without its problems, difficulties and dilemmas but it is all made a lot easier because everyone is working towards the same end and seeking to live the program.

The big tension for me as a faith community leader is between doing what I believe to be the right thing and trying to remain popular at the same time. What is right is not always popular and what is popular is not always right. There is a pressure to do things that are visible and seen so as to gain favour and those who feel obliged to contest the leadership are not slow to take advantage when there is an apparent lack of action in some area or another of the organisation's life.

There is always a pressure to seek the praise of people at the expense of conscience and there are difficult decisions that involve doing the right thing rather than just the popular thing. This has come to the fore in recovery as I am seeking to follow the will of God in situations rather than doing what is easiest and most popular.

9.22 Mr New

When I was a child there was a man who lived up our road called Mr New. He had been working as an expatriate in Kenya and then Japan. He was an expert in setting up whisky distilleries and that is what he had done in Africa and the far-east for many years.

When he had finished these assignments, he, his wife and three children started the process of moving back to their house in England. His wife came home first but it was clear that Mrs New had a problem with drink. Living the ex-pat life had taken its toll as had the endless supply of free alcohol. On arrival at her home in England, she fell asleep in the bath with her very young son and they almost drowned. One day she came round to our house in a terrible state and shared with my mum that she had incurable pancreatic cancer and that she had been told that she would be dead in a matter of months.

After she died Mr New had to return home permanently to look after the family but he also had a drinking problem and spent well over a year drinking all day every day in the local pub. One day he just stopped drinking and began a new life. It was so sudden and noticeable that we all remember it.

I don't know how it happened but he completely stopped drinking, got a new job and remarried. It was a remarkable turnaround and even though I was a young lad it made a lasting impression on me.

9.23 Hill Running

Although I can no longer do long-distance running, I can scramble up hills, so I do that. I live close to a steep escarpment that I have been using for training. Having set a target of five repetitions each session I found that I was lying to myself about how many I had done.

The solution to this has been to choose five small stones which I transport up the hill one day and down the hill the next. In this way, I can't deceive myself about how many times I have scrambled up the escarpment. It reminded me of how I used to deceive myself about my drinking. I had a wonderful ability to forget how many drinks I had taken especially if I was taking wine from a winebox.

This form of exercise has also been reinforcing one of my most important recovery behaviours which involve focussing on what's on the ground in front of me and not trying to look too far ahead. When I am scrambling up the hill I have to focus on where I am putting my feet because of the loose stones and unstable ground. It is easy to slip and fall down if I don't give the next step my full attention. The same is true on the way down because the hillside is dotted with rabbit holes and if I am not paying attention I can easily twist, sprain or even break my ankle. It's a lesson in not getting distracted and just focussing on the next step that is in front of me which is important not only in my hill running but, in my life, as a recovering alcoholic.

I need to pay attention to what is directly in front of me in life and not allow myself to become overly absorbed in the distant horizon of distracting thoughts which are way off in the future.

9.24 A Way to Go

Sitting in the car park outside my recovery meeting at a town church on a warm summers evening I could see and hear the loud and raucous banter that was going on as people arrived at the door. It was all very friendly and fun and it reminded me of a barroom scene from a wild west movie. I wondered what sort of church the people walking past thought that this was? It amused me because it was more like the doorway to a nightclub than a place of worship.

It was fun and alive but at the same time, it made me realise that in terms of the promised serenity of the program we may all have some way to go. Some of us are highly theatrical and like a drama, others are just loud and noisy whilst more than a few just sit outside the doorway chain-smoking. It's a sort of reality drink advert with no drink except tea. If this is what alcoholics are like on tea just imagine what we would be like on alcohol.

Despite the din, we are all a pretty well-behaved bunch who in spite of having a way to go in our recovery are on the path of progress. We have not arrived we are all a work in progress as we move forward from where we are. We all started in different places but there are many miracles of recovery and demonstrations of change amongst us.

The person laughing loudly could easily have been the person in the town centre drunk and screaming their head off. The person chain-smoking at the door may have just kicked a twenty-year heroin habit and a lifetime of addiction to alcohol. The alcoholic drama queen may have just escaped the horror of a seven-year abusive relationship where she was endlessly beaten. We all have some way to go but we are here, in recovery and not in the pub or the front room with a bottle of vodka and the curtain drawn

9.25 Losing Something

When I signed up to work for the church as a priest, I said to a friend of mine that I felt like I was losing something by going into full-time religious work. He was surprised at my comment because he thought it must be wonderful to have a vocation and to be able to fulfil it.

Before I went professional, I was carrying and transmitting my faith to the people around me and I enjoyed being part of that process. Because I was not being paid for this or seeking anything back from the people, I found that they were interested and wanted to hear what I had to say about God and my faith. However, as soon as I left my secular job and began to work for the church this element of surprise was lost and people expected me to go on about God.

I think there is something very significant in the way that twelve-step fellowships are committed to the principle of being non-professional. This doesn't mean unprofessional it just means non-professional. The absence of any sort of fees or payment to the organisation means that people coming into recovery people can know that you are not in it to get their money or anything else off them.

Recovery has come freely to me and I want to give it freely to others. It would be tempting to become an addiction recovery professional but I don't want to do that as I think I would lose something, just as I lost something when I went professional with my faith.

There are very few things in this life where you are offered something that is entirely free with no strings attached but strange as it may seem alcohol recovery through Alcoholics Anonymous is one of those rare commodities.

9.26 Amazing Grace

My understanding of Grace is that it is the empowering presence of God to enable us to be the people we are meant to be and to do the work that he has called us to do. Grace is God's work in us that enables us to rise above and move beyond our circumstances.

I believe that behind all the work that goes on in recovery is the unseen hand of the God of grace. Grace is the antithesis of self-effort because it is God doing for us that which we couldn't do for ourselves.

I am conscious that although I am cooperating with God it is by his grace that I am sober today. If my own willpower and self-control could have stopped me from drinking then I would not have needed God. However, seeing as all my own resources completely failed to overcome the power of alcoholism in my life, I have to acknowledge that it is by the grace of God that I have been set free. It is not my own doing because I couldn't do it.

John Newton wrote his famous hymn about this and described it as amazing grace. His words are worth repeating. 'Amazing grace how sweet the sound that saved a wretch like me, I once was lost but now am found was blind but now I see.' Later on, he wrote 'twas grace that brought me safe thus far and grace will lead me home.' Newton knew by experience the power of saving grace in his own life as I do in mine.

It is by grace that I have been saved from the power of alcoholism and the early death that it would have brought me had I carried on drinking.

9.27 Alcohol Will Find You

If you are a potential alcoholic you don't have to find alcohol, it will find you. Even in cultures where alcohol is banned people still manage to be alcoholics. How is that? As Bob Dylan said the answer my friend is blowing in the wind.

We just don't know, but what we do know is that alcohol seems to have an uncanny knack for finding its victims. Alcohol is on a seek and destroy mission and as potential alcoholics, we find ourselves as prime targets.

Monasteries, priest's houses, convents, churches, and religious sanctuaries of all flavours are no obstacle to the insurgence of alcohol. It's like those heat-seeking missiles that lock onto their target engines and blow them out of the sky.

Does all this sound too far-fetched and dramatic for you? I don't think it's far from the truth. Even when I was training to be a priest, I would go away for our residential training weekends and low and behold there would be a bar in the retreat centre. Even worse it would be an honesty bar with no one really taking note of how much drink was being consumed.

Lurking around every corner of my life was a bar, a drinks trolly or a small fridge with a mini-bar in it. It was a set-up all placed there by the enemy of my soul to trip me up again and again.

Make no mistake if you are an alcoholic, even if you are hiding from the stuff, it will find you.

9.28 Staying on Beam

I have moments when I feel that I am moving fully in the will of God. These times are generally fleeting but they are accompanied by a wonderful sense of freedom. I heard a song the other day that described this sense of freedom that is found in the centre of God's will. The lyrics were 'for its only in your will that I am free.'

When I'm in my will I'm subject to all sorts of limitations as I seek to get my own way. But when I'm in the centre of the will of God I find freedom that I get nowhere else. It's a liberation and a break from my bondage to self.

I guess the art of living skillfully and well in this world is about staying on the beam or as close to it as possible. It means making constant moment by moment corrections so as to stay on course. Like a plane coming into land when there is poor or no visibility. Survival depends on not going off beam and I have spent too much of my life going that way and paying the price.

I am seeking to constantly align myself to the searchlight and navigation beam of Gods Spirit that is always shining even in the darkness. I don't have to fly around in circles anymore looking for the runway because I have a guiding light who is the God of my understanding.

More than that I now have a much better idea of how to lock onto that beam and it's a great relief. Being on beam gives me a sense of freedom that only comes when I am aligned to the will of God.

9.29 More than This

My alcoholism has deposited within me a natural sense of dissatisfaction with the way things are. I want something more and I have the feeling that there must be more to life than this. This restlessness and desire for more are still with me even in recovery. I used to drink on it and it kept me drinking as I was demanding more and more from the drink in order to satisfy this craving for something more. I've heard it said that Alcoholism is a disease of more and this makes perfect sense to me as I feel a deep inner longing for something more.

The frustrating thing is that I don't know what it is that I'm longing for. I'm longing for something more, but what is it? I think the answer is not to be found in any material thing or human relationship. This desperate desire for more is I believe a spiritual dis-ease. This is what I am up against when this feeling is on me. I am wrestling with spiritual hunger and thirst that no can of beer, spirit or bottle of wine will satisfy.

St Augustine spoke of the God-shaped hole that only God could fill and satisfy. I believe he was onto something and I have a strong sense that the way forward for me when I feel like this is to turn my attention towards God. Deep down I know that if I direct this desire and hunger for more towards God then I will be able to find and experience at least something of the more that I am longing for.

9.30 Don't give Up

An alcoholic friend of mine used to love a song by Peter Gabriel called don't give up. The chorus says 'don't give up, don't give up, don't give up, cos you have friends.' It also says 'I believe there's a place, there's a place where we belong.' I too used to play this song a lot before I came into recovery. I suspect it may well come from the writer's own experience and struggle with depression.

The thing is that we can't do recovery on our own because we will most likely give up. Years ago, someone said to me 'the banana that leaves the bunch gets skinned.' What they meant is that I can't do this on my own. My natural inclination particularly when depressed is to separate and to isolate. In the past, I have run away and hid when I should have sought out the company of others. I am not meant to live on my own because when I do, I am vulnerable to my alcoholic mind and that gives my alcoholic thinking free reign.

Fellowship is more than a social club or even a church, it's a group of people who are bound together to help each other towards a common objective. In the case of alcoholics like me, that objective is to live a sober and useful life. I can't do this on my own but together we can make it.

Today I recognise when I am isolating and withdrawing from fellowship. It's quite a subtle process as I gradually drift off and out of sight. I am good at disappearing without attracting attention. When I realise what I am doing I have a choice. I can continue down the lonely and dangerous road of self-isolation or seek help. Help is there for me in the form of a raft of friends in my recovery fellowship who will be delighted to hear from me. They have the rope ladder and they are equipped to help me out of my hole.

This life of recovery is not a solo journey, it's a pilgrimage with many others along the road. Together we can and will make it.

October

10.1 Wine Boxes

I listened to a radio phone-in and the subject that people were being asked to chat about was wine boxes. It was very funny and amusing as people shared their techniques for getting the last drops of wine out of a wine box. In an entertaining way, the conversation revealed the desperate lengths that people would go not to miss out on those final few drops of wine in the bottom of the foil skin inside the wine box.

Whilst there was lots of humorous conversation about techniques to get all the wine out what was not discussed was why people were so desperate to get at those last few drops. It was assumed that everybody whom this affected was someone for whom this was of the utmost importance.

There was no mention of the fact that wine boxes provide a clever way to disguise how much you are really drinking. Wine on tap in the home is an ingenious idea and the fact that it's difficult to keep track of how much you have had until it runs out is an extra bonus.

From my own point of view, wine boxes were useful as they reduced the number of bottles that tended to accumulate at an alarming rate.

Not only were wine boxes less tough on the conscience, some of them even contained decent wine that was actually nice to drink.

10.2 The God of our Understanding

The recovery program that has facilitated my recovery from alcoholic drinking is an unashamedly spiritual one but it is not a religious one as it does not advocate any particular theology or religion. This has the effect of avoiding conflicts and arguments about God as well as preventing anyone from being excluded on the grounds of their particular religious beliefs or theology. It aims at achieving a working knowledge of God in practice rather than stuffing people's heads with a load of knowledge that bears little relation to life. I have always thought of it in terms of my car which I can drive without knowing how all the parts of the engine and gearbox work. What is important to me is that I can drive it so that it gets me where I need to go.

I have had to set aside everything that I think I know about God so as to clear the ground to experience him in my life, particularly my life of addiction. I need a relationship with God that works on the ground because without divine strength and wisdom I can't live a sober life. My PhD in theology will not stop me from picking up a drink, in fact, it could easily facilitate it if I allow my thinking to eclipse my living faith. I can reason and talk myself out of faith in God as well as into it so I have to be very careful with theology. My theology can be as toxic as alcohol for me so I have to be careful with it.

What I aim for these days is a real working knowledge of God especially in the form of connection and conscious contact. This is much more exciting than formal theology as I now walk-through life with God. I am not alone and I am not doing life on my own anymore. I am vitally connected to the God of my understanding.

10.3 Covering Up

As a priest, I have presided at hundreds of funerals and walked through the valley of the shadow of death alongside many families as they begin to process their loss. More than a few of these deaths have been caused by alcoholism although the link between the drinking and the subsequent death has not always been obvious. The death certificate may indicate things like cancer, trauma through a car crash or fatal burns as the result of a house fire so the actual cause goes unrecorded and hidden.

In trying to help arrange funerals and produce eulogies for bereaved families I have been struck by the way that most of the time no mention is made of the deceased persons alcoholic drinking that has brought about their early death. Not only is it not mentioned but it is avoided or completely denied as it is either cut out of their life story or minimised to the point of being a minor addendum to their life.

I have wrestled with this as I feel it is a cover-up by the family that prevents people even family members from really knowing the person who has died. At a funeral, I once made what I thought was a humorous comment about the deceased persons drinking but it did not go down well with the family. They wanted to keep up appearances as I guess they felt that it reflected badly on them. The irony was that I used to drink with him so I knew that he had died from this disease.

Alcohol has a good cover-up team rather like those CIA agents who clean a crime scene of all forensic evidence. Alcohol does the damage, kills the victim, covers up, blames someone else and then leaves the scene as if it had never been there.

10.4 Not a Course

Recovery is not a course where you finish and get a certificate or a medal at the end. The problem with all courses is that they eventually come to end and then what do you do? I love courses and I have taken many courses in different things all through my life but the problem for me has been that just as I am starting to really enjoy it and get into it the course comes to an end. I took a harmonica course once and just as I was getting the hang of it the course ended and I've never made any real progress since. In fact, because it finished and I had to stop going, I have lost most if not all of the skills and knowledge that I acquired on the course.

The same is true of many alcohol recovery courses that do a good job helping people to understand and even break with their addiction but when the course finishes there is no longer any support and relapse is almost inevitable. The same dynamic is a play in some rehabilitation courses even residential ones. They are excellent for the duration of the stay but once the time comes to leave what then? Unless there is support at an individual level then it's a tall order to expect ongoing recovery especially if life gets tough as it inevitably will.

The reason that I was so glad to find Alcoholics Anonymous and its program is that it never finishes or comes to an end. There will always be a meeting to go to or a person to call for help. Sponsorship provides one-to-one instruction and support and the sponsors' office will rarely be closed or the phone turned off. The hand of fellowship is there for me twenty-four hours a day.

Courses are as good as they go but they don't go far enough for me which is why I need the program, meetings and a fellowship which is always there for me and will always be there for me. It never ends or finishes.

10.5 Self-Pity

I am not a big fan of my own self-pity because it is so destructive for me as an alcoholic. Feeling sorry for myself and wallowing in self-pity is not a good idea because I know that ultimately it leads to a drink.

As with a lot of character problems I find it easier to see self-pity in other people than I do in myself. I particularly notice it in my fellow alcoholics in the early days of recovery. As with all of us on that journey out of addiction we produce a litany of excuses for our drinking that are often rooted in self-pity.

As I help people in the detoxification phase of their recovery, I often hear the all too familiar refrain 'if you had my life then you would drink' or 'if this had happened to you then you would drink.' Many of us in recovery have indeed experienced genuinely terrible circumstances in our lives but no matter how bad they were they are all poor excuses for continuing to kill ourselves with alcohol.

The 'poor me' attitude is not a very attractive one and rarely secures the real help that we need to climb out of addiction. The antidote to self-pity that is promoted in all situations of recovery is gratitude. Gratitude takes our focus off ourselves with our apparent lack and redirects our gaze outside ourselves to what we do have as well as what we have to give. What we have might not be much compared to others but it is a start.

I remember being at a recovery meeting and going for a coffee with a recovering alcoholic after the meeting. He produced from his pocket a tattered piece of paper which was his gratitude list. It was humbling to listen to him read it out as he had so little compared to me or indeed most people. He was truly grateful for all that he had been given in his newfound sobriety and there was not a sniff of self-pity as it had been sent running by his genuine gratitude.

If I do find myself descending into self-pity, I don't hang around in it anymore. I get out of it as soon as I can by practising gratitude and helping someone else so as to take the focus off me, myself and I.

10.6 Reaching Out

As I see people drinking recklessly in town centres as they are carousing and off their heads on booze, I want to reach out and help them, but I can't. There might be exceptions to this but as a rule, they can't be helped until they reach out for help. Tough as it may seem that's the way it works with alcoholism. It was true for me and it is true for them because nobody was going to criticise or challenge my drinking. It was my right to drink the way I wanted and I didn't want any do-gooders coming round telling me how to live my life.

However, walking past these still suffering alcoholics in the park or the doorway of a derelict shop I can't help thinking where their rock bottom might be. How low or desperate will they get? Will they ever come into detox and recovery or are they the unlucky ones who are on a one-way ticket? There are miracles of recovery but sadly many never find the healing and redemption that they so desperately need.

I found myself describing a group of street drinkers as 'alkies' but then I realised what I was doing by using this word. I was setting myself apart from them and drawing a distinction because I wasn't on the street. But I have the same disease and it is only by the grace and mercy of God that I am not sitting with them drunk. There is no room for snobbery in this business of alcoholism.

When I walk past my fellow alcoholics, little do they know that I am one of them. I say to myself 'there but for the grace of God go I' and I pray for them that they might reach out for the help that they need.

10.7 Just Feeling It

Today I'm not doing anything to change the way I feel. I don't feel comfortable in my own skin. There is a sense that something is just not right in my inner being. I know this state of heart well and I don't like it. It is exposed because I am not using things, substances or people to blot it out. When I experience this, I sense that I am face to face with the roots of my alcoholism.

I am just allowing myself to feel and experience my life as it is. I am not running away into some distraction or habit to change the way I feel, but instead, I'm just sitting with it. It is very uncomfortable but I do know that as people often tell me; 'This too shall pass.' I also know that by staying with it and not trying to escape these feelings I am learning things about myself and my disease that I could not access in any other way. In the past, I would have run away from this discomfort into many different forms of escape such as exercise, compulsive working, obsessing about objects and things that I want to buy, and of course drinking.

Now I am seeking to ignore the urges to run and being still I can identify the things that come to me as I sit with these feelings. This is healing, spiritual healing and it is not in my power or guided by my hand. I am putting myself in the hands of a power greater than myself so that he can skilfully and carefully perform the necessary soul surgery.

10.8 Investing in the Connection

My new neighbour has just moved in and the first thing he has done is to have the pavement dug up so that he can have a faster and better internet connection. His priority before doing anything else is to establish a good and effective connection and he has invested a lot of time and energy into making it happen.

His investment in improving his connection got me thinking about my connection with my higher power that for me is God. I can't just dig up the road and connect to God's fibre optic network because it doesn't work like that. How it works for me is that I give time and energy to meditation and prayer so as to establish a good and stable connection with God.

It is not easy but it is possible if I put the work in. Daily times of being still and quiet, augmented by spiritual reading and prayers. It's a fairly simple approach but it works and I find that from this short time spent daily in these practices I can go on to enjoy days where I am increasingly conscious that I have a connection with God.

This is not the exclusive preserve of priests or religious people but is open to everyone. There is no set blueprint for our connection to a higher power as everyone is wired slightly differently. I want to continue investing in this connection with my higher power, my God.

10.9 Staying Put

One of the most difficult things to do in recovery can be to just stay put. As I have got better, I have wanted to change my location. Every time I have been seriously tempted to do a geographical, I have found myself being blocked. I have sensed my higher power, my God saying just stay, don't move.

The picture I have in my mind is of a father with a child on the other side of a busy road. Everything in the child is urging him to run across the road but the father is shouting just stay there, don't move.

I am where I am for my safety and for my recovery which takes time. I'm in the right place but my illness wants me to place myself in situations where I can't cope and where it can once again take advantage of me.

I can feel like that young child wanting to respond to my inner urge to run but as with the child if I act on that impulse I may well get run down. When it is time to go then my God is more than able to communicate when, how and where I am to go, but until I have that information I will just stay put.

Being in the place I am meant to be is my place of safety and that's why I am staying put.

10.10 Busy Head

Like a lot of others who struggle with addiction, I have a busy head. There is just too much going on in my mind and this makes it difficult to focus my thinking.

Tasks like studying become impossible because there are too many distracting thoughts going on at the same time.

A friend of mine who used to use heroin described how the drug would just blank out all the overwhelming flood of busy thoughts in her mind so that she could have some temporary peace.

Many of us find at least in the early days of our drinking that alcohol does the same sort of job. It shuts up our busy heads so that we don't have to think. For a long time, alcohol had the effect of unplugging my overloaded mind as it turns 'the thinker off.'

Of course, alcohol and drugs just provide a temporary fix and the busy head returns often with even more to think about as the effects of the drink wear off.

10.11 Groaning in Prayer

In recovery, we are encouraged to pray but the question is just how do we do this? There is no easy answer but there are some pointers on how to direct our prayers. Arrow prayers sent up in emergencies do I believe have a place and maybe they have saved some of us from some pretty dire straits.

Everyday life can be challenging and I guess a good prayer for anyone in recovery is 'God keep me away from the first drink today.' Of course, I have to actually want to be kept away from that drink and take every appropriate action to avoid it.

What I am trying to do when I pray is the will of God so that my prayers line up with what he wants to do. What I am trying to avoid is telling God what to do. I don't believe that my prayers should be a sheet of instructions or a to-do list for God.

Sometimes I don't have words for what is in my heart to pray. I think at such times God is putting in my heart the things that are on his heart and I may never be clear about what they are. These prayers are more of a groan or a weight in my heart.

The important thing is that I am available and placing myself at God's disposal to serve his purposes. Most of the time I don't see the results or the effect of my prayers however there are other times when there is an obvious or fairly instant result.

Recently I had a few hours to kill in a town centre and I prayed a prayer something along the lines of 'have you got anything for me to do here.' Very soon after praying that prayer, I met someone who knew me and really needed to talk something through urgently. I was thrilled that God has put me in the right place at the right time to meet that need simply because I was available.

Prayer changes things not necessarily in the way I want them but even if I can't see it at the time Gods responses are always for better in the long run.

10.12 Never Better

One of the things I have learned in my own life and seen in the lives of my fellow alcoholics is that when we are drinking things never got better and in fact, they only get worse. The day I put down the drink and sought help with my recovery my life started to get better. Life took a turn for the better and instead of things continually going wrong everything started to take off.

It really was an extraordinary turnaround as my life began to get better. Things started to work out for me in ways that I could never have thought possible. Good things started to come to me without my having to strive or fight for them. Blessings seemed to be poured out in a way that I had not been open to before.

This was all because I was going in the right direction instead of going the wrong way down a one-way street. Drinking is a one-way street for alcoholics because life only gets worse and never better whilst we are pursuing our drinking careers.

I was amazed at how much better I felt after even a few weeks of not drinking. Mentally I started to recover and I noticed that my sense of humour had returned. It was if I had put a new pair of glasses on and things looked so much clearer and better than they had before.

I can easily forget how bad it was as I now enjoy a good life without alcohol. I have hope and a future now that I am no longer drinking myself into an early grave. Life has never been better for me as I am finding healing and increasing release from the disease of alcoholism.

In the past I could not imagine a life without alcohol now I can't imagine one with it.

10.13 Drinking to Forget

I used to drink so that I could forget everything. I wanted to blot everything out by getting out of my head. I wanted to forget my cares and worries and the only way I could do that was to get drunk. That was the one time when I could just forget about everything and let go.

Of course, when I came round nothing had changed and things may have been worse but at least I'd had a break from what I felt to be the relentless pressure of life. As long as I was able to drink, I could just about keep ahead of things, especially the past, but if I stopped then I had to deal with life and I could not imagine ever doing that without a drink.

So, I was trapped by the past and my need to forget about everything. It seemed to me that some temporary respite was better than no respite at all. Getting drunk provided that relief but unless I was drunk my past was always there, on my back, reminding me of all my failings, faults, weaknesses, and personal defects. I was permanently in the dock under a barrage of accusations that I had no defence for.

My faith was supposed to take away the guilt and shame but I could not seem to get it to work for me in this way. I was stuck and I could not let go of the past. All I could do was blot it out with alcohol.

It's only been as I have got unhooked from my past that I have been freed from the urge to drink to forget. I don't forget the past but I have come to terms with it and been putting it in order the best I can. I am not constantly plagued by flashbacks or moments of terror as some memory is triggered and brought to the forefront of my mind.

I no longer dwell on my past but neither do I have to blot it out with alcohol anymore.

10.14 Knowledge and Wisdom

In recovery, I have been given knowledge about my true condition as an alcoholic. Perhaps the single most important fact for me is the knowledge that alcoholism is a disease, not a moral failure.

Having this knowledge is one thing but doing something about it is another. If I am to make use of my knowledge, I need wisdom. This is why the recovery prayer or the serenity prayer as it is called, asks God for wisdom. It's a prayer for the wisdom to be able to live the right way on the basis of the knowledge that I have received.

There are loads of intelligent people who are hooked on all sorts of substances including alcohol. They might start to understand their addiction intellectually but wisdom comes when that knowledge is put to work and actively applied to the problem. Wisdom arrived for me when I took the knowledge that my alcoholism is a disease and applied that knowledge to the problem by stopping drinking.

More than that I applied wisdom to my knowledge by attending recovery meetings and getting involved in a program of recovery so as to deal with the underlying problem. My knowledge tells me that this is an incurable disease and wisdom directs and moves me to act on this knowledge by staying actively involved in the program of recovery that has brought me lasting freedom from alcoholism.

When I was drinking, I had knowledge about many things but I didn't have the wisdom or indeed the power to live in the light of that knowledge. In recovery I live much more wisely than I used to, primarily because I now pay attention to my higher power, that is my God who is directing me and keeping me on course in my daily walk through this life.

10.15 Distortions of Reality

I have to be careful about my perception of reality. As an alcoholic, my perception of a situation can be very distorted. In my head, I can picture a situation that doesn't exist in reality. An alcoholic friend of mine recently described to me how his perception of his marriage was that it was over and that he and his wife would have to get a divorce after fifty years of marriage. When he explained this to his wife she just laughed and burst the imaginary bubble of catastrophe thinking that was all in his head. He had read too much into his wife's behaviours and come to a ridiculously distorted view of what was really going on which was all in his alcoholic imagination.

These experiences are the bread and butter of my alcoholic mind even when sober. This is why my fellowship with other alcoholics is essential as they are often the only ones who can blow the whistle on my distorted thinking.

When I sense that I am getting a distorted perspective on any situation or relationship I take a reality check with those people in recovery who I know will see through my faulty thinking and prevent me from making foolish and rash decisions based on false perceptions of reality.

10.16 Beautiful People

In recovery, I meet people who like myself would not be described as 'the beautiful people.' Most of us have been pretty beaten up and have the scars to prove it. Many of us have done ourselves a lot of damage so to the casual observer we are probably far from beautiful.

However, there is another sort of beauty that I see in the rooms of recovery and it's a beauty that transcends our normal ways of seeing. In recovery, I meet people who carry an inner beauty and serenity that is almost magical. There is something about recovering alcoholics particularly as we gather together that transmits a love and compassion way beyond the norm.

I have never felt more loved and more included anywhere else and the love that I feel emanating from others is tangible. It is the most extraordinary phenomenon made all the more remarkable because of the circumstances by which we have all been brought together.

As I go on in this fellowship of recovery, I feel the love more and more perhaps because I myself am getting deeper and deeper into the recovery process and the program. What I have come to see is the tremendous good that is in all of us if we are encouraged to flourish and thrive.

Our program works relentlessly on the negative aspects of our characters but what we may miss is the way that as the silt is polished away, we begin to shine. Like diamonds, some of us have had some deep cuts but they mean that we can shine even brighter because although often in heavy disguise we are 'the beautiful people.'

10.17 Thinking Straight

What I have discovered in recovery is that so much of my alcoholic problem has its source in my thinking. I can now see that I was very headstrong when it came to my thinking about drinking and this spilled over into many other areas of my life. These days I am not so self-assured and I am more circumspect about asserting my will as I am far more questioning of my own motives.

I remember my father coming home fuming from a cocktail party where a psychologist had challenged him to examine his motives. I can still picture him wandering around the house in an absolute rage saying over and over the words 'examine my motives who does she think she is.' In retrospect, I think that this lady hit the bullseye as she managed to get through to my father in a way that few people were able to do. Of course, it is a good discipline to examine our motives and it is one that I practice as part of my recovery program.

One of the things that I do now that I would never have done in the past is to ask God to direct my thinking. Even with my faith prior to coming into recovery, I was firmly in charge of my thinking. It was my mind, my thinking and that was my department. Without realising it I was very closed-minded because I was not open to the idea that the God I believe in might actually be able to direct my thinking better than I could.

I am still working on this every day as my own best thinking comes into contact with ideas from the mind of God. In the past, I have treated his will as an opinion to go into the melting pot of ideas so that I could make an informed choice. I was placing myself in a position of absolute authority and complete autonomy over my thought life. In this scheme of things, I was the managing director and God was just an ordinary member of the board with a voice and a vote.

Slowly I am learning that things go better when I let God take his place as chairman of the board in my head.

10.18 Looking for Connection

Behind my alcoholism is a deep need for connection. I am looking for connection with other people and with my God. When I was drinking with people, I would often feel really connected to them and it felt good at the time. This connection was not only short-lived but, in a way, it wasn't even real because it was chemically induced and therefore not truly authentic.

I know why people take ecstasy at dance venues because they want to feel that connection with the people in the room. It's a powerful feeling to be connected with others through alcohol and drugs and I know from experience the sense of spiritual communion that comes at such times. Sadly, this experience is short lived and there is a price to pay in terms of hangovers and withdrawal from chemically induced euphoria.

These days I find the connection that I have been looking for amongst others who like me are walking out of addiction. There is something unique about recovery fellowship in terms of the level of communication and communion that is there for anyone who wants it. I guess it is partly a function of people sharing their stories and being absolutely honest but there is something more.

There is a bond and fellowship of suffering that enables the deep connection that I and many other addicts have been looking for in all the wrong places.

10.19 I Was Wrong

Admitting that I was wrong both privately and publicly is very humbling and therefore difficult to do. Hard as I found it to accept, I have had to admit that I am an alcoholic and that I have been wrong about my drinking habit. It was all wrong from the beginning because I should never have taken alcohol into my system in the first place. I can make excuses and there are reasons why I did this but at the end of the day, I have to say that it was wrong for me to drink alcohol.

As I have admitted privately and then more recently publicly that I have been wrong about my alcoholic drinking it has opened the door for me to admit that I have been wrong about many other things. I have had to take a big dose of humility as I have confessed to being wrong about a lot of things both at home and at work.

This has not happened all at once but gradually I have noticed that the words I was wrong, have been coming out of my mouth on a regular basis. As long as I hold onto my ingrained desire to be right about everything I am in trouble. I don't know why I didn't catch onto this earlier in life although I suspect that my unwillingness to admit that I was living wrongly with drink held me back in other areas when I should have just put my hands up and said I was wrong.

The great thing about this is that it is so liberating not to have to defend a lie. It is so freeing to live completely in the light and not to be covering anything up or pretending that everything is alright when it is not. True confession is both powerful and liberating despite being initially very painful and humbling.

10.20 Alcoholic Loneliness

It is only as I have come into recovery that I have realised just how lonely I had become in my drinking. The alcohol cut me off from everyone including my wife and family. I felt very alone and the fellowship that I craved, I just could not find.

That was until I came into recovery and discovered that there were loads of people just like me who also experienced deep loneliness whilst craving fellowship. At first, I only found this sense of fellowship in a diluted form and it wasn't until I got more actively involved that I started to really feel it as I began to lose my deep sense of inner loneliness.

I still have times when I feel very alone even with people around me but I find that if I connect with the fellowship in some way then the loneliness tends to lift. Why it is that other alcoholics should provide this when others can't, is a mystery to me. I don't understand it but I know that it works and that's the important thing.

What this means is that if I want to limit my sense of loneliness then I need the fellowship of other alcoholics who can help me as no others can to rise above my alcoholic loneliness. It might seem obvious but it took me a long time to realise that I can't break free from loneliness by myself.

10.21 Entirely Ready

I have begun to see that I was not able to find release from alcoholic drinking until I was entirely ready to let it go. Before that, I would want to let it go when things were bad but when life improved, I would want to pick it up again. I had not really let go even though I thought that I had.

Entirely is an important word for me because it sums up neatly the position that I had to get to in order to quit drinking. I had to be entirely ready, not nearly ready or almost ready, or sometimes ready, I had to be entirely ready. I had to really mean it deep down inside and not just pay it lip service.

What I am describing is what I would call getting to the end of myself. I came to a point where I had to admit defeat. I could not find a way to hold on to my drinking as well as holding onto life. It was one or the other. I had to make the decision to really stop and get help or carry on and face a very uncertain future of decline, loss and early death.

I wanted to have my cake and eat it. I wanted the benefits of not drinking whilst still being allowed to drink. As long as I hung onto a thread of an idea that I could perhaps, maybe, one day drink again then I was not entirely ready.

It was only when I was able to say to God, okay I am ready, take it away I don't want anything more to do with alcohol that I was able to find freedom from the compulsion and the mental obsession to drink.

10.22 Choosing What is Right

In sobriety, the power of choice returns and I am faced with decisions that involve choosing what is right and avoiding what is wrong. I am face to face with the responsibilities and dilemmas of choosing my pathway in life. Alcoholism is a never-ending series of wrong choices all stemming from the bad decision to pick up a drink. It was a bad decision that I made over and over again but I just kept on doing it as my will was firmly rooted in the decision to drink.

I made bad decisions and poor choices as I pursued my selfish ambition to drink. Instead of making decisions that were based on what was best for me and for those around me I learned to make decisions on the basis of what I wanted to do, which was to drink. My need to drink came first. Even if it wasn't obvious to others or even to me at the time, drinking alcohol always held a high priority. It was always a priority as I needed to drink.

So, I was willing not to do what I knew to be the right thing in order to be able to get myself the kind of drinking that I wanted. Drinking like this is a very selfish way of life and recovery has involved breaking this cycle of selfish behaviour where I make poor decisions and choices based purely on self.

I still find myself being tempted and pulled off track by my own selfish desires and the schemes that flow from them. There is a battle of wills as my will goes head-to-head with my higher power, who is God. I know when I am pushing in the wrong direction and when I am deliberately choosing to go the wrong way but it's amazing how powerful this delinquent urge is within me.

When I get fixated on something that I want, the obsessiveness of my alcoholism kicks in and I can't let go of the idea however unrealistic or destructive it might be. At such times I find myself on the front line between right and wrong. I am all too aware of my alcoholic propensity to choose the wrong and ignore what is right so that I can get what I want.

However, in recovery and with this awareness, I now have the power of choice and those choices are more often than not, the right ones.

10.23 Changing Rooms

I have exchanged the barroom for the recovery room. In the recovery room, I can stay and change or I can leave. In the barroom I can stay, not change and never leave. The minute I go back to drinking all progress ceases and all positive change comes to an abrupt halt. By way of contrast, every minute spent not drinking and actively involved in recovery is a time when positive change is taking place in my life. In recovery, I am not going backwards but instead, I am moving forwards and changing for good.

Change for me now is a process of letting go of my old ideas and saying yes to the directions of my higher power, who is God. Daily it is about giving more of myself over to the purpose and plans of God rather than seeking to run the show myself. As the captain of my own destiny, I was just piloting the ship onto the rocks as I desperately sought to control the circumstances of my life so that I could get through. Every morning I now hand my will and my life over to this power, this supreme intelligence who is far greater than me and is able to provide me with safe passage through the rocks and shifting sandbanks of life.

On the estuary near where I live large ships have to take on board a pilot who takes the wheel and steers the ship up the constantly changing narrow passage between the shifting banks of mud and sand. The old charts are of little use because the waterway is always changing and last year's route will no longer provide the necessary depth for the huge hulls of the container ships.

My old patterns and charts for life are no longer fit for purpose and like the ships I too need someone to pilot me, I need somebody who knows the way through. Not only does the pilot set the overall direction he also makes numerous mid-course corrections and adjustments to account for the tide and currents. My life in recovery is like this as it has not only required a complete change of course and direction but it is also subject to moment-by-moment adjustments and changes in order to keep me from hitting the rocks or getting stuck on the sands of life.

10.24 The Fantasy Factory

I think that I lived in a good deal of fantasy even before my drinking took off. At school, I was obsessed with the music culture and used to live in my own imaginary world that was fuelled each week by the New Musical Express.

Some children dream of being famous footballers or even footballer's wives but my dream was to be a

Rockstar. It seemed to me to be the only real option in terms of a career. I imagined that it would be a life of excess with a healthy diet of sex, drugs and rock and roll and of course no real work. When I did eventually venture as a drummer into the world of rock band's I found that the reality was very different indeed.

Behind the fantasy was the idea that if you wanted something badly enough you could get it and that there were no limits to what you could achieve if you wanted to. At one point in my city life, I had a boss who used to tell me very forcefully that I had to think big and that if I kept my big ideas to the fore then I could only succeed. Needless to say, he was an alcoholic too.

The reality was of course far different as I found it increasingly difficult to get out of the pub let alone put legs on my big thinking. I was into big drinking and the big thinking would only come on stream somewhere between four and five pints. These alcohol-induced fantasies would never involve me doing any work or having a particular aptitude or talent. In my mind, it would all just happen as I would be catapulted effortlessly into the limelight as I walked out of the bar.

Reality is tough and fantasy is one way to mentally cope but in the long term, it is not a good solution. The dreams that I have now are grounded in reality as they are no longer inspired by alcoholic fantasy. Importantly they are no longer entirely self-centred as in recovery my focus has been continually shifting towards helping others.

These days my daydreams are realistic and very often they are directed towards bringing joy to others rather than putting me on some sort of pedestal.

10.25 Terminal Alcoholism

Alcoholism is an incurable and fatal illness that has killed some of my best friends. They have all died of this illness without ever understanding what was wrong with them or being able to do anything about it.

This disease has one particularly lethal twist and that is its ability to convince the sufferer that they haven't got it or that it doesn't exist. Even those like myself who find recovery are not out of the woods because even after decades of sobriety we can relapse and the results are usually pretty catastrophic.

People who are suffering from terminal alcoholism are not bad people they are just very sick. In fact, they are often brilliant people whose company you would enjoy and whose presence you would miss. But the fact remains that the disease of alcoholism is a progressive one that never gives up on those who have it. As in my own case, it can lie fairly dormant for many years but it has not gone away.

In the last couple of years, I have lost two of my friend to alcoholism. One died of cancer caused by alcohol and the other hung himself. Untreated alcoholism is a terminal disease and there is no known cure. What there is and this is what is keeping me sober is a well-tried program of recovery that provides an antidote and as long as that treatment is maintained the disease can be kept at bay.

However, many of us have a tendency to think that we can beat it on our own and we strike out on our own program. Occasionally it might work but for the great majority, the result is usually further relapse and even greater powerlessness over the disease which eventually leads to an early death. Every day, I have to keep in the forefront of my mind the fact that for me to drink is to die.

10.26 Doing my Own Thing

It is not that I don't know the will of God for my life it is just that I don't want to do it. I have a much clearer idea of the pathway laid out for me than I like to admit.

Following God's will for my life is only difficult because I have an alternative set of plans. These personal plans involve doing things that are off-piste and usually dangerous to my spiritual health and sobriety.

Why do I harbour such deviant desires, hopes and dreams? I don't really know for sure but I am fairly sure it is connected to my alcoholism. Left to my own devices and doing my own thing will only lead me back into chaos but I still deliberately choose to make my life as difficult as it can be by departing from the script that has been given to me. I want to do it my way and that usually flies in the face of God's way.

As a friend of mine says sometimes I have the spirit of stupid. It just comes on me and I go off on some hair-brained scheme that at best ends up going nowhere or at worst lands me in a load of trouble.

Life goes so much better for me when I stop trying to do my own thing and get in line with God's purpose, plans and ways.

10.27 Two Interpretations

Every situation in my life has at least two interpretations and the main ones are mine and God's. When I am facing situations in life, I am asking myself how am I going to see this and how am I going to handle it? Am I going to see this from God's perspective or mine? How am I going to interpret what is going on? Am I going to see this situation as God at work or has everything just gone wrong?

In recovery, I have interviewed for a couple of jobs one of which I was offered and the other I wasn't. I didn't actually end up taking the job I was offered because I felt that it just wasn't right. What I did was that I accepted it and then I felt increasingly uneasy about it as I came to realise that I had gone after the job because it was gratifying to my ego. It was a much more high-profile position but in my heart of hearts, I knew it was wrong so I pulled out.

The job that I didn't get I now see from God's perspective. At the time I was upset as I felt rejected and not good enough. It wasn't even a particularly high-profile job and more of a sideways move motivated partly by my desire to live closer to my ageing parents so that I could look after them a bit better. My interpretation of that event now is that God knew my motives, he also knew what the job would bring me in terms of trouble and difficulty and he prevented me from getting it.

Both of those positions would I believe have compromised my recovery and they would also have precluded me from continuing my PhD studies which I now know I was meant to do. As I have had time to reflect on these two situations my initial interpretation of these events reflected my disappointment and a certain loss of face but now, I can see the hand of God in this as he protected me and guided me into the right path.

10.28 Changing on the Inside

Recovery for me is about my ongoing agreement to engage in a constant process of positive change in my life. It is a daily decision to say yes to the challenge to become the person that God created me to be.

The process of change that I am engaged in through recovery is what I would call deep change. This is the type of change that starts on the inside first and then works its way out into my life as it impacts the way that I live.

Of course, there is resistance to change within me and that's why I need the continual help of the program with my higher power behind it. I don't always want to change because I have got so used to living in a certain way that feels familiar and safe. I don't want to change track but change I must if I am going to keep sober and sane in the long term.

Change is not all bad and not as bad as I thought it was going to be. In fact, it makes life much more interesting and there are always further challenges that help to keep me changing for the better.

10.29 As I See It

The perceptions that I have of my situation in life can be very distorted and often out of focus. In recovery, I have become much more open to looking at my circumstances from different angles in order to try to get a more accurate picture of what is going on.

I have also been taught that I am less able than I thought I was to untangle my personal web of feelings and thoughts without help. I am in need of other people who are also on this journey of recovery to help me because they too have been travelling the same pathway. Many of them are way ahead of me and this can be very useful as I seek the way forward in life.

Self-understanding is the name of the game here as I get insight into what is really going on inside of me. Why am I feeling like this? Why is this situation making me feel so resentful or angry? How come I allowed that to happen again?

These are the kind of diagnostic questions that I have been taught to ask in recovery as by seeking to answer them more light comes into my situation. I don't always get immediate understanding and instant revelation but often the answers do come if I stick with the questions.

These all make for a more interesting and nuanced life than I had before. There is a feeling of growth and excitement about the future as I make new discoveries and get fresh insight into life.

10.30 Baffled by Circumstances

In my life of recovery, I hit up against situations that baffle me. These situations usually concern relationship issues in which I am unable to understand what on earth is going on. Instead of launching into a tirade of blame and criticism of another person I now hold the mirror up to myself and ask what my part is in the situation. What am I bringing to the table here?

There might not be an immediate answer or a lightbulb moment but I know that I need to sit with it and as I do the answers will come. I am not only baffled by situations but also by some of my reactions and emotions that arise from them. Why am I feeling so resentful about this? Why am I struggling to accept this situation? Why do I want to run away? Why is this person living rent-free in my head all the time?

The answer is always out there and often it is outside of my control. What I can do is to clean my side of the street by looking to see if I am trying to control the situation or negative emotion in some way. It is only when I do this that I find the light begins to dawn, I can gain understanding and then not be so baffled by the circumstances.

10.31 Stuckism

I don't want to be the same person that I was last year, last week or even yesterday. I don't want to be forever stuck in the same attitude or patterns of negative and destructive thinking that have dominated my life through alcoholism. I want to break free from these chains of negative perceptions and thoughts that have controlled my life.

I have spent too much time stuck in the repetitive cycle of destructive drinking to want to continue in other destructive patterns and cycles of living. Every situation of difficulty both in myself and outwardly in life is an opportunity for me to get unstuck from the negative patterns and reactions to life that I have inherited and developed in dysfunctional environments.

I don't want to remain stuck in these behaviours or patterns of thinking. I can break free as I work my program and call on a power greater than myself. Recovery is about finding new ways of living so that I don't have to remain stuck like an old vinyl record playing the same groove over and over again. I am no longer a stuckist and stuckism no longer appeals to me.

November

11.1 An Inside Job

Changing my job, my life, my appearance, or even my wife will not change me. I made many different changes to my way of life when I was drinking in order to try and control my alcoholism but none of them worked in the long run because they didn't deal with the real problem. Changing my external habits and patterns of living does not change me.

Deep change does not come from the outside in but from the inside out. I have found that real and lasting change is an inside job. My change from being an active to a sober alcoholic began on the inside. I don't even really understand it but something happened inside me at the deepest level of my being that brought about an inner shift and it was this change of heart that ultimately brought me sobriety.

The external changes were a manifestation of the process of transformation in my inner being. For years I had been trying to change myself from the outside in. A strong cocktail of different routines, new disciplines, and alternative patterns of living could not change the fact that I still wanted to drink.

The external method of change could never get to the heart of the matter because deep within I was still holding on to alcohol. This is where the deep change needed to take place because I needed a complete change of heart as well as a total change of mind in order to break free.

11.2 The Heat is On

The heat is on as my life gets busier and fuller in recovery. It's a wonderful thing to get my life back from the domination and tyrannical rule of king alcohol. But now life is hotting up and I am finding myself under intense pressure in both my work and home life. This is the real test of my sobriety and my program.

My circumstances are placing me way outside my comfort zone and my familiar patterns of life. In the past, I would have leaned on the bottle to get by but now I am finding other ways through. The main guiding principle for me today is the slogan 'easy does it.' People around me are also under pressure, some are panicking or giving way to fear.

As I am tempted to get caught up in the atmosphere of nervous anxiety, I am just repeating this slogan over and over again. It is calming me down and preventing me from making stupid mistakes due to panic or through losing my nerve. The heat is on but I know that if I take it easy and don't give way to fear I will be alright. This too shall pass and in a few days everything will be alright.

It is at times like this that my recovery program really kicks in. In a very practical way as it is helping me to live in the moment and not to give way to even the thought of taking a drink.

11.3 Happy as I Choose to Be

I am increasingly conscious of the weather that I carry as I engage in my daily encounters with those around me. What spirit am I carrying to the people with who I am interacting every day? Am I projecting a positive and encouraging spirit or am I broadcasting a miserable, depressed and negative persona?

Alcoholism tends to breed negativity and it is easy to end up just oozing it from every pore. One of the unwritten rules of the bar that I used to attend was that you were never under any circumstances to let on that you were happy about anything. The tone of the conversation was always subdued, cynical, bitter and generally the polar opposite of happy. In fact, if Mr Happy had appeared at the bar he would probably have been forcibly removed.

Now that I am walking in freedom from the shackles of alcohol, I am allowed to be happy. I have taken to allowing myself the possibility that I can be happy and the strange thing is that I do now experience moments even days where I would say that I have been happy. I am obviously not deliriously happy all the time but I do enjoy happy days and happy hours that are very different from those that are advertised outside of bars.

What I have realised is that happiness is a choice and it is not necessarily tied to everything going well or being just how I want it to be. I can be happy at a funeral, not because I have no feeling for the deceased or his family but because I carry happiness in my heart that is not entirely dependent on circumstances.

I can in fact choose to be happy because happiness is a choice and not something that I have to deny myself unless I want to.

11.4 Acting Out

I have been deeply infected with the 'if it feels good do it' philosophy that was part of the post-1960s zeitgeist as I was growing up. This combined with active alcoholism meant that I sometimes found it very difficult to take action that was contrary to my feelings. I had handed over far too much power and authority to my feelings so I could feel great pressure to obey them even when my rational self was saying that I should resist the temptation to 'just do it.'

What I have been learning in sobriety is to pause and not to obey the urge to act out of my feelings. I now have the ability to say no to myself even when my feelings are calling to me and pushing me to act out. I no longer have to go along with my feelings and I can deny myself in ways that I just could not do before I found recovery.

I have had to grow and develop in this as it didn't happen overnight and I still have to constantly check myself in this arena of life. I find that particularly with strong feelings like fear I can act out by immediately reacting to situations where it would be better to withdraw and work through the feelings so that I can not just react but respond in the most appropriate way.

I no longer have to act out of fear or any other intense feeling that wants to take me over. My feelings can be very intense so I have to be careful but I know that as long as I am not taking in alcohol then I am much less likely to give way to the urge to act out and I am far more inclined to respond in an appropriate way.

11.5 Staying on God's Side

I used alcohol to change the way I felt and for a long time, it did help me to deal with life and the problems that I experienced each day. However, I knew deep down that I was on the wrong track. When I was using alcohol in this way, I knew in my heart of hearts that I was not on Gods side. It was as if I had stepped over a line and I was giving my life and my energy to another power.

When I was using the drink in this way, I had the sense that instead of being on Gods side I was siding with the enemy of my soul. I wanted to be on Gods side but because of the drinking that I felt compelled to do, I found myself on the other side of the street. I wanted to be on Gods side but my drinking put me in opposition to God.

The reason for this was that God loves me, he wants to best for me and he would not let me get away with drinking in this way because it was diminishing the life that he had mapped out for me. In recovery, I can now choose to stay on Gods side of the street in all my affairs including but not limited to alcohol.

At every turn of the day, I have choices and there are decisions to be made. Am I going to stay on Gods side of the street or am I going to cross over and do it my way without him? Am I going to live as a friend of God or am I going to join the opposition and live as his enemy?

Now that I am free from alcoholic drinking, I can stay on Gods side and know his favour and blessing in all my activities.

11.6 Taking My Will Back

To pick up a drink would be for me to take my will back. I would be saying to myself and my God that I want to do it my way because that is what I want. I now know that this is folly and will only end badly but the desire to go my own way is still there. It whispers to me and suggests certain courses of thought and action that would completely sabotage my recovery.

Ultimately, I would find myself being drawn away from my connection with God and find myself being led back into confusion, chaos and eventually drinking. My will is strong and once I get fixated on a thought or idea then I find it difficult to let it go. I know from experience that in such circumstances the best thing I can do is to get myself to a recovery meeting because it is there that the answers usually come. Very often someone will share something from their own experience that gives me the corrective that I need. I get light and then peace.

I can arrive at a meeting very troubled by a situation especially one where the assertion of my will is the problem, only to find that by the end of the meeting the problem has just gone. It was all in my head and I have been fighting a phantom.

At other times it is a process of letting go of my will and allowing the situation to unfold without my control or domination. Recently I refrained from acting on the impulse of my will and God stepped in and the problem was wonderfully removed. If I had acted out and tried to fix it myself in accordance with my will it would have caused a lot of trouble. By handing it over and leaving it there I was able to see my higher power work in a marvellous way that wasn't just best for me but for everyone else involved.

11.7 Recovery is Not a Theory

Recovery has come to me through taking action not sitting around thinking about it. I was brought up and then educated to seek to understand the theory first and then to apply it to my life. I have found that this does indeed work in many areas of life but not in recovery from alcoholism.

Recovery is about doing and taking action not just thinking and theorising. I have to do recovery and that requires action on my part. My recovery has continued to gain momentum ever since I acted on the thought that I should go to Alcoholics Anonymous. I had the thought, looked up the meeting time, caught a train and showed up.

It was there as a result of taking action and going there that I started to hear the things I needed to hear that have enabled me to find sustained recovery. I have since studied some of the theory and continue to do so as part of my recovery but the real progress comes to me as I do it and live it.

Recovery is not a theory it has to be lived and it is as I live it that I start to get the fruit of a sober life.

11.8 Marinated in Fear

Growing up in an alcoholic home meant that I was marinated in an atmosphere of underlying fear and tension. My father's fear was expressed solely in terms of anger which would be bubbling away under the surface of things. My mothers fear and anxiety came out in different ways mostly through obsessive cleaning with bleach and very bad psoriasis all over her body.

My father's fear was rooted in his childhood where he had nothing, not even enough to eat, and so it was not surprising that material security, especially freedom from want, was the highest priority for him. The only time I saw his fear expressed in any other way than anger was after he survived peritonitis following an emergency appendectomy. I remember him in the hospital bed after the operation and when he saw us gathering around his bedside he burst into tears. I was pleased that I saw that as it showed me that my dad was only human and it reminds me not to judge him because he was just as vulnerable and afraid as we were.

Constantly living in this environment meant that I unconsciously soaked in the family fear and the tension that surrounded it. My mother's anxiety also added to the emotional marinade in our home and I absorbed it into my being as a child. My fathers fear and my mother's anxiety created the perfect emotional soil for my own alcoholism. I was set for a fall even before I had taken my first drink.

I was thoroughly marinated in a potent mixture of anxiety and fear that like a loaded gun was just waiting for the trigger to be pulled, which of course it was when I first took two shots of vodka.

11.9 Getting Out of the Way

In the past, I have tried very hard to do things entirely in my own strength. I have operated as if everything depended on me and my wisdom or skill. What I am learning in recovery is that I don't have to cross all the t's and dot all the i's. Instead, I am exercising faith in my higher power and his ability to do something about it. This might involve me taking some action but often it involves me just leaving it with him.

It might sound easy but actually, it is harder than you think. Knowing when to act and when to step back is an art. It requires a lot of self-control as my instinct is to get involved or to rush in to fix the problem right now. What I am learning is that I don't need to take over from God as if he can't manage without my intervention.

Many things work better for me if I don't try to fix them myself. This is not laziness or neglect, it is more a recognition that God can really be trusted and if I rely on him and listen to him, then all be well. In fact, many of my difficulties arise from getting involved in something where God is already at work, taking care of it.

All I really need to do is to fully trust him and get out of his way whilst he takes care of it for me. This is faith in action and it really works.

11.10 Like a Moth to the Light

I went into the kitchen and turned on the light only to hear the repetitive soft thud of a moth banging its head against the window. It was totally desperate and absolutely frantic to get in the kitchen as it was being driven crazy by its craving for the light. Thankfully the window was closed and I shut the blinds to cut out the light. The moth stopped its headbanging and disappeared into the night.

If the window had been open it probably would have succeeded in its quest and would have destroyed itself by repeatedly banging itself against the hot light bulb until it was mortally wounded.

The moth reminded me of a thirty-nine-year-old friend of mine who died a few days ago from the effects of alcoholism. Like the moth, she could not keep away from her obsession that in the end caused her death. She knew it was killing her but it kept drawing her like a moth to the light. She just had to do it and she had to go back for more and more until her broken body fell to the ground.

Whilst we are engaged in active alcoholism that is what we are doing. We are bashing our heads and our bodies to pieces not on a hot lightbulb but with the contents of bottles and cans. To the outside observer, this is crazy but to active alcoholics and moths this makes perfect sense

11.11 Drinking Aftershave

A few years before I came into recovery, I used to go out running with the son of a friend of mine. He was in his early twenties and had not long been out of detoxification and rehabilitation for alcoholism. On these runs, he used to share with me some of his experiences with drinking and the one that really stuck in my mind was his emergency admission to the hospital following his drinking a bottle of aftershave. He had been so desperate for alcohol that he had taken to drinking a bottle of aftershave which had badly burned his throat and he was in a lot of pain. At the time I thought this was pretty crazy but now I know that he is not the first nor the last to try this solution to deal with the craving for alcohol.

On those runs, he used to share other things and without him knowing or me realising it I was identifying with a lot of his alcohol-related war stories. As he shared, I found myself thinking I've done that as he told of some embarrassing things that he had done whilst under the influence. He didn't know that I was an alcoholic and at that point in my life neither did I. He had just asked me to teach him to run but he unwittingly taught me about my alcoholism.

Thankfully this young man has maintained his recovery and sobriety and I am hoping that one day I will be able to tell him how he was used to initiate the process of my waking up to the seriousness of my own condition with this disease. Hopefully, I will never have to drink aftershave or any other poison in the compulsive and obsessive quest for alcohol.

11.12 The Ship of Fools

Alcoholism is not new it's been with us since we started to crush grapes. In the old story of Noah and the flood he gets out of the ark, plants a vineyard, makes wine, gets drunk and then disgraces himself.

In medieval times the church took little action against drunken priests although there are records of them being thrown out of the cities and towns. In Germany, the persistent alcoholics were rounded up and the city authorities paid merchants to put them on the so-called ship of fools so that they could be taken downriver to be dumped somewhere else.

In the early twentieth century in the USA alcoholics were forcibly committed to insane asylums often by their own families. Thankfully by the Grace of God, there was a mutiny in 1930s America when the ship of fools found a way to help themselves. The fellowship of Alcoholics Anonymous provided a new vessel that did not remove people from their families or homes but helped them to support each other where they were.

I am so thankful for this ship of fools because without it I doubt that I would have been able to maintain my sobriety. It's free, it's local and it works! In every town and city, the ship of fools is permanently moored up waiting to receive those who have had enough of getting more and more sick with the disease of alcoholism.

11.13 Declaration of Dependence

I hasn't been until recently in my recovery that I have really begun to value dependence rather than independence from God. I was always holding something back just in case and by holding on to some level of independence, I was not quite giving my all to God. I guess I could not totally trust God to look after me and therefore I needed to keep something in reserve.

I was holding onto some measure of self-sufficiency just in case God didn't come through for me. I could not quite let go and trust God for everything so I had to have backup in place. I would put together a plan 'B' in case God's plan 'A' didn't work out or work out the way I wanted it to.

My independence has been deeply rooted in my lack of trust and has held me back from fully realising all that God wants to give me. If my hands are full of my own resources then there is not room for me to receive what God wants to give to me.

I need to tear up my declaration of independence and replace it with a declaration of dependence on God in all things.

11.14 I'll Get That

When my good friend Frank was at the bar in my local pub, he would never let me buy myself a drink. As I ordered the next pint a cry would come from the other end of the bar as Frank would shout 'I'll get that.' Frank was a binge drinker who would appear in the pub periodically and exhibit great bar room generosity as if he were a millionaire and that money was no object. I'm not sure how he felt about it the next day as he looked at his empty wallet and nursed his horrific hangover but I was grateful for the crumbs off the masters' table.

I now think of the phrase 'I'll get that' in relation to God. In recovery, I am finding that there is a provision that I never found when drinking. Things seem to fall into place in a way that just didn't happen when I was in active alcoholism. I have a new experience of Gods favour in my daily life that I never thought possible. It is as if God is saying 'I'll get that' when some need arises and I don't have the resources to take care of it myself.

Recently God has provided for me in a most wonderful and unexpected way that is beyond my wildest dreams. In fact, I had thought that this particular financial liability would be with me for the rest of my life but very quickly, unexpectedly and miraculously it has been lifted from me. It's as if God has raised his voice from the heavenly bar room and said 'I'll get that.'

11.15 Consequential Losses

Alcoholic drinking has consequences and these manifest in material, emotional, psychological and spiritual losses. My alcoholic mind suffers from a strange twist or blind spot that finds it difficult to give sufficient thought to the potential consequences of alcoholic drinking.

In most other areas of life, I am a rational, cautious and sensible person but when it comes to alcohol, I do not immediately connect the idea of drinking with the potential negative consequences. When the compulsion to take a drink was on me, I would brush aside all other rational and sensible thoughts in order to get myself to the drink.

How is it that as an alcoholic I can pick up a drink with the full knowledge of what the potentially disastrous consequences will be? How can I throw all caution to the wind for the allure of alcohol? The truth is that I don't know the answer to this. All I know is that when I sit down after the event and analyse it, I can see that I was foolish and selfish and that I was prepared to override my reason and common sense just to get drunk.

I am now aware of this strange twist in my thinking and I am prepared for it because I don't want to go down that road again. I know that drinking is front-loaded as it offers me an almost irresistible instant hit and uplift. I have to be aware of its insane call and I cannot afford to pick up the first drink even though the chorus in my head is saying 'go on it's only one drink.'

The consequential losses for me have been heavy. Not so much materially but emotionally, psychologically and spiritually. There is an emotional and psychological price to pay for alcoholic drinking in terms of depression, low mood, anxiety, fear, paranoia and negative thinking. Spiritually there is an intense shame and a large amount of guilt to fend off as well as a sense of separation from God.

Thankfully, now that I am not drinking these losses have been largely reversed and I am free from their effects as long as I can have the presence of mind and the power of God behind me to say no to the first drink.

11.16 Traction

I knew my faith was important and powerful but what it didn't seem to possess was traction with my alcoholism. No matter how much energy I put into my faith it did not enable me to find the freedom that I needed from alcoholism.

I tried Bible studies on addiction and loads of recorded talks on the subject. I tried healing meetings with the laying on of hands and the anointing of oil. I spent a lot of money to attend a church in Toronto in the hope that I could find release in their meetings. I went to deliverance sessions to see if I could get the demon drink out of me but it had no obvious effect.

I knew that my faith did work and should work but I could not get it to work on my drinking. Nothing worked for me and sooner or later I would always end up drinking again. I am sure these things did help me and there were some significant moments when I could feel some sort of shift or release but it never lasted.

It was not until I started attending Alcoholics Anonymous that my faith started to gain traction with my alcoholism. As I got over my religious prejudices and let go of my theological stumbling blocks, I started to access the power of the twelve-step program. Rather than contradicting my faith, it encouraged me to earnestly seek my higher power and to improve my conscious contact with God. It was these things that I saw demonstrated in the lives of other alcoholics who has found the necessary traction between faith and recovery.

Since coming into recovery my faith has been activated and empowered to do what it always promised to do, which was to liberate me from every destructive power and enable me to live a really useful and faithful life.

11.17 Small Steps

Recovery for me has been comprised of many small steps that didn't seem that great at the time but each one has contributed to a steady and solid recovery from alcoholism. As I look back over the last ten years, I can see that I have made a continuous series of small but good decisions that cumulatively have resulted in a life that is taking me in a much better direction.

Unlike drinking the results are not usually instant and they take time to manifest themselves. It's not that I have a lot more possessions or that my circumstances are easy but what I have been given is the gift of gratitude and appreciation for even the most simple of things.

I would say that in recovery my life has been truly blessed day by day as I have sought to live the way that I am being directed by my higher power. I had some good people in my life before recovery but the difference is that now I appreciate them and I am grateful for them.

Step by step I have come to appreciate all that is good in my life instead of always focusing on what I perceive to be wrong or lacking. I now see that recovery is a process of step-by-step growth that is almost imperceptible but over time amounts to a significant amount of positive change.

11.18 Workaholism

A lot of my alcoholic energy I invested in my work as a vicar. Instead of drinking alcoholically, I worked alcoholically. This involved constantly overworking and focussing all my energy on the parish. The consequences of this were not good for me or my family. I was preoccupied with work as I was thinking about it so that I was often emotionally unavailable to my wife and children.

My ministry took precedence over everything else and I gave it a top priority. Like alcohol I let work take over my life and it was all done in the name of God. Time and again I would put work first just as at other times I put drinking first. It was the same process and pattern that I used in my drinking.

I was using work to fix me just as I had used alcohol, but it didn't work. I didn't achieve anymore and through overworking I was probably less effective than I could have been if I had taken a more balanced approach.

Having quit alcohol, I have to watch my workaholism because it tends to creep up on me as I find myself obsessing about work and work-related situations. The key for me is balance and moderation which for an alcoholic is the holy grail of mental capacities.

11.19 Living on a Spiritual Basis

My life is now on a different footing as I live on a spiritual basis. My recovery from addiction is not based on psychological or physical techniques but on spiritual principles. This is the thing that so many of us alcoholics kick against. We don't want any of that God business we just want to get rid of the trouble that drinking is bringing us.

Some of us aren't that sure we want to give up alcohol entirely and we are not convinced that we have to. What has God or a higher power got to do with drinking anyway? The answer is quite a lot as my alcoholism is a manifestation of a spiritual malady. It is a symptom of my soul sickness and my need for something more.

Without getting to the spiritual roots of my drinking problem all other treatments will only be symptomatic ones. They might cover over the underlying disease for a while but eventually, it will break out in a new form if the primary infection is not being treated.

Living on a spiritual basis is not a one size fits all program but a bespoke pathway placed in front of us by our higher power. There is a way out of addiction for each of us, should we choose to take it. It is a spiritual path not a religious one and it involves a personal connection with a power greater than ourselves. That power has the map and the compass. He knows the way from where I am to where he wants to take me.

It is a spiritual pathway and there are many alcoholics like myself who have found it to be the only permanent way out of this affliction.

11.20 The Wolf in Sheeps Clothing

I've been walking past an old inn that has been a place of hospitality for over five hundred years. It's a pub complete with a log fire and a barroom that always looks so inviting. At night all the bottles are lit up and I am finding myself drawn to it like metal to a magnet.

It all looks attractive and welcoming. It's so natural and normal. Could this really be a potentially dangerous place for me? What harm could I possibly come to in a lovely old country pub like this? The answer is that despite its apparent harmlessness it is for me a place of danger.

It is like a wolf in sheep's clothing as at one level it is just a lively, friendly place of hospitality that broadcasts easy conviviality and for most people, it poses no threat or danger. But for me, this old inn is a place where I need to be alert and cautious. In a place like this with its innocuous and benign charm it is easy for me to get lulled into a false sense of security. It's the sort of place where my alcoholism starts to reassert itself. It starts suggesting to me that I am taking this alcohol business too seriously and that if I just relax and maybe even have one small drink them everything would be fine.

For most people, the old inn is a great place to go but for me, as a recovering alcoholic it is a risky place to be however nice it looks from the outside. Like a casino or the races to a compulsive gambler, this is not a place for me to relax my guard. I can't afford to take any chances with it however inviting and innocent it seems.

I have to remember that for me alcoholic drinking however beautifully packaged is just a wolf in sheep's clothing.

11.21 Last Orders

Last orders in the pub were always a scramble to get the last round in as we approached drinking up time when the landlady would cry time ladies and gentlemen, glasses please. This was all part of the ritual and the liturgy of pub life and we all knew just where we were with it.

Then everything changed and licensing hours were relaxed so pubs didn't stop serving drinks after lunch and they never seemed to close often until late into the night. Off license sales were greatly relaxed with petrol stations selling alcohol twenty-four hours a day. Suddenly the external discipline of the licensing hours was removed and the temptation to stay later or drink for longer grew stronger.

External pressures will never stop an alcoholic from drinking but what the licensing laws did was to put some very useful boundaries in place that helped me when I was trying to control my drinking.

Prohibition of alcohol sales in the USA proved that alcohol will always find a way out no matter how much you try to control it. However, whilst it can't be outlawed, its sales and distribution can be regulated. Of course, alcoholics will always find a supply somewhere as securing a supply is the great obsession of every true alcoholic.

11.22 Closing the Gap

There was always a gap between myself and my higher power created by alcohol. I didn't know why God seemed so distant especially when I had given my life over to serving him as a priest. It was true that I had once experienced God's presence in powerful ways but these sorts of encounters were less frequent as my life went on and my experience of God was not consistent.

I had no idea at the time that this was connected to my alcoholism. I never appreciated the spiritual impact that drinking was having on my relations with God. It is only after finding recovery that I have realised what a gap I created with my drinking. I knew there was a distance but I never connected it with alcohol.

It had me in its power so that it eclipsed the sunlight of Gods Spirit in my life. Alcohol exerted its unholy influence but God was there even in the dark times. He withdrew and kept his distance until I was willing to really let go and ask him in to clean house.

The gap is now closed and I don't need to open it up again. These days I so value His presence that I go out of my way to avoid even the slightest of gaps. I now listen and obey God rather than the bottle.

11.23 Miniatures

At the age of eleven, I remember being really excited about being bought a bottle of Grand Marnier by my father. We had just eaten a Grand Marnier crepe from a street food stall in St Tropez. This was not a large bottle but a miniature and it was the start of my miniatures collection. This must have been a sign for the future as I was captivated by them. I was drawn to them and became an avid collector of all sorts of miniature bottles of spirits.

How strange that they should have such a captivating effect on me. I can still recall how thrilled I was when I was given a new one for my collection. Was this just a meaningless coincidence? Maybe it was for it proved to be an omen for what was to come.

Later in life, I could never understand why shops sold miniatures until an alcoholic lawyer friend of mine explained how they fitted neatly into his pocket so that he could have a couple of double vodkas on his way into the office.

Another alcoholic friend explained how she found it easier to justify her drinking to herself if she bought really small bottles rather than big ones. What I have come to realise is that for some alcoholics, miniatures form a small but important part of the psychology and practice of alcoholic drinking.

11.24 Anonymity

The idea of anonymity is an important for me as the notion of the alcoholic in the popular mind is an alarming one. Nobody wants to be labelled as an alcoholic because of the negative connotations that come with it. When it comes to working and having a professional reputation being known as an alcoholic or even ex-alcoholic can have a negative impact on jobs and careers.

So, the advice is to keep our heads down and not to blast news of our alcoholism from the housetops. At the same time those of us who like myself have escaped the clutches of the bottle have a strong desire to tell of our miraculous release. It's only natural to want to share the good news.

What the practice of anonymity does is to protect me and all with this disease from the alcoholic tendency towards self-promotion and the desire to make a name for ourselves. Even though we want to hold stadium meetings to tell people about our deliverance we have found that it is better, in the long run, to keep our heads down and get on with the work of recovery both personally and through helping others to find and sustain recovery.

My alcoholism is not a secret but I have to take responsibility for who I share this with and how.

11.25 Getting Away with Nothing

I think my teenage underage drinking set the stage for the idea that I was getting away with it. By getting served beer at a pub when I was clearly underage or finding someone who would buy alcohol for me, I felt that I was getting away with it and it added the sense of forbidden pleasure and excitement to the drinking. This sense stayed with me in the following years and when I was drinking, I felt that I was getting away with it or getting one over on some imaginary other.

I guess the most obvious way this idea manifested was in sneaking drinks at parties and social occasions or even at home. It's easy to get all sneaky and selfish about drinking. At the end of the day, it was only me who I was deceiving because I was the one who was paying the price.

Even today when I am in drinking situations, I notice people sneaking drinks. I am alert to how quickly and how much they are drinking. I watch people getting a sneaky chaser in as they order the next round in the pub or the person who is rapidly taking full glasses off the drinks tray as it is being passed around.

As I did, they think they are getting away with it but of course, they are not getting away with anything. Alcoholic drinking is a form of self-deception because ultimately, we have to pay the price. The tab will eventually come to our table and we won't get out before we pay in full.

11.26 Battling the Bottle

I never fully conceded victory to alcohol. I had not given in to it but what I did do after some major defeats in my fight with the bottle was to call for reinforcements. Like many of us, I had been trying to fight it on my own and I was just getting driven further back. I needed help and it came in the form of Alcoholics Anonymous as many friends gathered around me and drew me into their fortress.

Outside the camp, I was being ambushed and I didn't stand a chance. Alcohol had me pinned down in my trench and there was nowhere left to go. I was under attack from this enemy of my soul who wanted to destroy me. Out on my own, I had less and less to give in terms of the fight. I know why people give up the fight and surrender to the bottle. I had to get to the point where I knew that I just could not fight it anymore. Only then was I able to accept the solution that was being presented to me.

For most of my life I didn't know what I was fighting. I knew it was something but it was only in the last year of my drinking that I realised my true enemy was alcoholism and the awful power behind it.

11.27 The Hiddeness of God

I do have a fairly consistent sense of Gods presence these days. It took me a long time to get the hang of this but in recovery I found myself waking up aware that my higher power who I understand to be God was just there. I love waking up with a sense of His presence and peace and I tend to linger when this happens.

I can't turn it on or turn it off but I have learned to recognise and appreciate it. One of the things that have helped me to understand this is the idea of hiddenness and manifestation. Sometimes God is hidden and other times he manifests his presence. That seems to be the way it works and now I know this I don't fret when I can't sense Him and neither do I get over-excited when I know that he is with me in a powerful way.

What I can do is to put myself in the right place and position to experience Him. There is a worship of the heart, a mystical union and consciousness of living in the blessing of the father's love. Feeling it, experiencing God in the heart and having an awareness of Gods loving presence. It is about allowing God to love me.

God is in my heart, not just the head or my mind. It is the most wonderful and valuable thing in the world to know Him and His presence in my life. It is more valuable than anything money can buy. His nearness to me and my dearness to Him, whether hidden or manifest, I am sold on this.

His Spirit is so much superior to the alcoholic one that used to eclipse God in my life. Nearness and dearness.

11.28 Carrying the Can

I see more people than ever walking around cities and towns holding onto a can of beer. As I watch them it is like a visual aid to me that reflects the absurdity of the way I was holding onto alcohol and putting my faith in it. Instead of putting my faith in God, I was putting my faith in a liquid that I was clutching onto for dear life.

I find it much easier to put my faith in something that I can see or taste rather than in something that is unseen like God. It feels more secure and I feel safer when I can hold onto something physical rather than something immaterial and spiritual. Holding onto a bottle or a can seems so much more real than seeking to hold onto a higher power who doesn't have a label or cork.

The transfer of trust that has taken place in me has meant that I have had to let go of a physical substance and replace it with a spiritual one. Alcohol was all front as it delivered a fairly swift hit and made its presence in my body known in a tangible way. The new spiritual energy that I now have is altogether different because it is not front-loaded. It is subtle and its presence doesn't shout. It is fluid but not a fluid. It moves in unseen and unexpected ways and it always brings blessing rather than cursing.

When I see someone holding onto a can of beer, I think about how blessed I am that I have found a better way and a more reliable power to hold onto. A kindly and loving spirit who is out for my good instead of the alcoholic one that was seeking to steal, kill and destroy.

11.29 Controlled Drinking

When my children were younger, I used to speak on church ski holidays as a way of enabling my family to go skiing at an affordable price. I knew that on these trips I could not drink because I was aware that if I did there was the potential for things to go badly wrong. In order to pre-empt any embarrassment, I practised a form of controlled drinking which for me meant zero alcohol.

I can't remember making a conscious decision to do this but I think that deep down I just knew that I could not afford to drink at all whilst on these holidays. Interestingly I wasn't so physically dependent that I couldn't stop drinking for a few weeks but it wasn't controlled drinking so much as delayed gratification. I knew that when I go back home, I would once again have the opportunity to drink the way I wanted to and without anyone judging me.

I was also helped by the fact that it was with a group of people who were not drinkers in fact quite the opposite so that made things easier. However, even though I wasn't actually drinking it didn't stop me thinking about it because the mental obsession was still there. I would watch people in the mountain top restaurants as they drank with impunity wondering what the Swiss wheat beer tasted like.

My controlled drinking was a strange form of torture and a masochistic form of enforced abstinence based on the promise of future indulgence. On the outside, it looked like everything was under control but on the inside, my disease was building like a hurricane poised to strike land.

11.30 Take Fun

I was in my forties before I learned to ski. I wasn't prepared for all the falling over and clumping around in big boots or trying to carry skis to lifts. Thankfully I had a wonderful ski instructor who latched onto my need to relax and take it easy in the learning process. He basically had two instructions for me which were 'take speed' and 'take fun'. Take speed meant that I needed to go faster and take fun meant that instead of trying so hard I should focus on enjoying myself.

The idea of enjoying myself as I was learning to ski as well as savouring the experience of being in the mountains was not something that I could allow myself to do. I was focused on becoming a brilliant skier but the more I tried the worse I seemed to do with it. I had missed out on the fact that the whole thing was meant to be fun. I would never make the Olympics or even a black ski run for that matter but fun was an option if I could take it.

Taking or having fun is not something that I allowed myself to do and I think this goes back to my family home where the focus was always on work and working. Relaxing was considered to be slacking and there wasn't any concept of play or relaxing together as a family. Our early lives were task-orientated and purpose-driven with a focus on paying the bills and making money. The only exception to this was in the matter of drinking where alcoholic fun was allowed and encouraged. Early on in my life, I learned that the way to have fun was to drink alcohol and to drink a lot of it.

This scripting has proved to be difficult in recovery as I have struggled to know how to have fun in ways that do not involve alcohol. Having fun and enjoying ordinary life seems like the forbidden fruit for me, and in recovery, I still find it difficult to know how to 'take fun'.

December

12.1 We are Sailing

My life before recovery looked externally alright but internally, I was often battling a squall. It was like a sailing dinghy struggling to gain control in a strong and unpredictable wind. Through recovery, I am much more stable and I am less prone to suddenly jibe and knock everyone out of the boat.

This doesn't mean that I sail through life unaffected by the storms that come but I am much more secure and less likely to react in dangerous or damaging ways.

I enjoy watching people sailing their boats skilfully as it reminds me that through following my program, I too can keep on an even keel even if the weather turns stormy and life gets tough.

I don't have to react and capsize the boat anymore. I can keep the boat upright and stay on course even in the most difficult of conditions.

I value the gift of mental and emotional stability that has come to me in recovery.

12.2 Doing or Knowing

Before coming into recovery, I was committed to the idea that before doing anything I needed to understand it. Through going to Alcoholics Anonymous I realised that if I wanted to find lasting recovery from alcoholism, I would have to set aside my best thinking and just do what was being suggested to me.

It became clear that I needed to act first and then the understanding could follow. What mattered was not my understanding of the program but the fact that if I practised its principles, it would enable me to stop my alcoholic drinking.

I meet people who want to argue with me about the program and they tell me that they think there is a better way, so I just ask them how is their program working out for them? The answer is almost always that they are still drinking.

As an alcoholic, my thinking falls short when it comes to alcohol. I can think rationally and clearly about many things except alcohol. My best thinking never achieved anything of significance as far as my alcoholic drinking was concerned.

Although I have gained a lot of insight into my alcoholism, I still don't fully understand my drinking but what I do understand is that as an alcoholic I must not pick up a drink one day at a time, and if I don't, I can't get drunk.

I don't need a PhD to figure that one out!

12.3 I Believe in Miracles

In the last year, I have seen some miracles in the lives of those closest to me. I believe that these miraculous changes are in some way connected to my recovery. They are tokens and signs of the hand of God in my life as a recovering alcoholic.

It is as if God is righting my wrongs and straightening out my past in a way that I never could. He is undoing the damage that I have inflicted on my nearest and dearest as their hearts and minds have undergone deep and rapid transformational change. There is a favour and a grace in my life that I never experienced whilst I was tied to alcohol.

It is as if God is smiling on me and those around me as I see them being blessed. I have been searching for a smiley face pin badge to wear on my jacket because I want to express and celebrate the smile of God that is shining on me these days.

I believe that the change that God has brought into my life and the lives of my loved ones through my recovery is nothing other than miraculous. I believe in miracles.

12.4 Getting Mad

The link between anger and madness in the expression getting mad is a helpful one for me as it accurately describes what used to happen in our family home when my father was angry. His anger would be expressed in shouting, cursing, and blaming accompanied by a sense of intimidation and violence. He would literally go mad. Our house could be a frightening place to be for a child because there was a madman on the loose.

He could not control his anger once it kicked off and it was as if a grenade had been thrown into the house as his latest devastating and destructive anger bomb would explode all over us. Because we were standing right next to him, we were the ones who got caught up in the explosion. At such times our lives became centred around his mad internal world of emotional confusion, rage, fear, chaos and despair.

I too suffer from alcoholic anger but instead of it exploding outward it implodes. My reaction to my own anger is to suppress it and turn it in on myself. Outwardly there are no explosions and I seem calm, but on the inside, I am shouting at myself. I take out my anger on myself but it is just as damaging and destructive as if it were taken out on the household furniture.

My upbringing meant that I never learned to recognise or process my anger in appropriate and safe ways. I thought that I was not an angry person but I was just not in touch with my true self. I got mad in a different way as I sucked in all my anger, denied it and then used alcohol to dissolve it. Like everything to do with alcohol, this was only a temporary solution and my pile of anger and resentment just got bigger.

Now in recovery, I am able to identify my anger and then let it out in appropriate and non-harmful ways. I don't internalise it or push it down anymore but instead, I use it as a diagnostic tool that I can mine for information about what is going on in my mental and emotional life.

I look for the root of my anger so that I can deal with it. Like a rotten tooth it needs treatment otherwise it keeps breaking out in painful infections from below the surface. Root canal treatment can be painful but it stops the development of further infections. I now acknowledge my anger and deal with it early rather than letting it painfully fester and infect my life.

12.5 Searching for My Fathers Love

Alcoholism makes it very difficult if not impossible for others to connect with us and they can feel completely unloved as we pursue our obsession with alcohol. It's hard for children to understand why their father chooses to prioritise his drinking over them. A wife cannot comprehend why her husband chooses to spend his life with alcohol rather than her.

As the adult child of an alcoholic, I know that my fathers' disease meant that he was unable to give me the love, approval and emotional security that I needed. He provided generously and self-sacrificially on a material level but he was not free or able to really love me as his child. I think he wanted to but just could not do it. I don't hold it against him because I know that he was suffering from undiagnosed and untreated alcoholism.

What I have realised in recovery is that throughout all my adult life I have been longing for, looking for, and trying to search out that love and approval that my father was not able to give me. Like a ship driven against the rocks, I have become wrongly tangled up with people from whom I desperately tried to get this love and approval but these folk were always unable to give it to me.

Time and again I sought out people who I hoped would be able to offer me the love and emotional connection that I was seeking with my father. I was drawn to people who were like my father and of course, they too were dysfunctional people usually alcoholics from whom I would try to gain some sense of love, approval and emotional security, however faint.

I now know that this need will probably never be entirely satisfied by any human being because they are not my father. More than ever, I turn this hunger for my fathers love over to my higher power that is my God. At the end of the day, it is only my heavenly father who is able to supply this higher love that I am so hungry for.

12.6 More Punishment

Alcoholic drinking is an extreme form of self-punishment. Day after day the dreadful cycle of drinking takes its toll on the body and mind of the sufferer. It's a strange form of self-torture that ends up killing us in one way or another. If you really love yourself or even just like yourself it is difficult to imagine engaging in the relentless process of self-destructive drinking.

The irony is that most alcoholics would not treat other people the way they treat themselves. We would not do this to other people because we know that it is not the right way to treat a person. Yet we do it to ourselves.

In the last year, two friends of mine have destroyed themselves and died as a result of their alcoholism. Both of them hated themselves and their lives so they practised self-neglect and self-abuse to the point where their bodies gave out.

No one could help them because they had agreed with the lie that they were no good and that they did not deserve to live. They looked back at the carnage of the past and gazed into what seemed to be a hopeless future and decided that the best way was out.

Not everybody can shake off the oppressive yolk of self-hatred but those who make it in recovery are those who are able to develop a new and more positive sense of self so that they can have real hope and a future that they want to inhabit.

Knowing that my alcoholism is a self-destructive habit that has its roots in self-hatred and low self-worth helps me to honour myself and to constantly seek a way of life that builds up my self-esteem rather than destroying it.

12.7 Denial, Acceptance and Change

It wasn't so long ago that my young nephew asked me a direct question in front of my mother. He said to me 'did your father hit you?' My mother was right there and he had put me on the spot. Normally I would have deflected the question but I was cornered. I said one simple word and that was 'yes.' At that moment I was dragged out of denial. It was very significant as I admitted in front of my mother and my family that I had been physically abused by my father.

I would not want to have called it abuse and I still don't like the idea of having to put that label on my father who I love and respect but it is the truth. For so much of my life, I have denied this and refused to accept the truth that I was an abused child. Having come out of denial I have moved into a place of acceptance and I have been open to receiving the healing and the help that is available to me.

This acceptance of the truth is bringing change as I can now after all these years start to move on because I am no longer stuck within and acting out from my childhood abuse. I have been able to accept myself in a way that I couldn't before as I had been blaming myself all my life for what had happened to me. I didn't blame my father for the abuse. I blamed and condemned myself for what had happened because deep down I believed it must be my fault or the result of something that I had or had not done.

My denial about this childhood abuse, my dyslexia and my alcoholism have all been linked. Coming out of denial and into a place of acceptance about my alcoholism has opened the door for me to be able to break the barriers of denial in other areas of my life so that I have been able to begin to find real and lasting change in those areas.

I have a sense that this process is not yet finished as the tight grip of denial is continually being loosened and released.

12.8 Human Experience

Somebody reminded me yesterday that we are spiritual beings having a human experience, not just human beings having a spiritual experience. I now live on a spiritual basis because I believe that I am a spiritual being as well as a human one.

When I used to live on a purely material basis, I was very confused about myself and this world that I live in. It was my ongoing spiritual malady that brought me into recovery from alcoholism. It took me many years to come out of denial and into a place of acceptance about this disease but I now see this struggle with alcohol as a part of my own spiritual pathway and journey into life.

I do not regret the past because I see it as God's preparation of my spirit for a future life beyond this one. I see this life of human experience as a training place for the real-life that is yet to come.

My human experience of life has I believe been designed and tailored specifically for me. I do not see the tough times and struggles in addiction as a bad thing as they have been used by God to sculpt me into the person I am today.

I know that I am not just a body or a mind but a real person with a spirit that is eternal. That spiritual flame that is my spirit is alight and aglow in a way that it has never been before. My spiritual life and my recovery are united and are all part of my development as both a spiritual and a human being.

Through the process of recovery from alcohol addiction, I am more aware than ever that I am a spiritual being having a human experience.

12.9 Discovering Self Respect

One of the main casualties of alcoholism is our self-respect which goes into terminal decline in direct proportion to the amount that we drink. Alcohol gives a temporary boost to our sense of self but it is illusory and short-lived. When the effects of alcohol diminish, we are left struggling to hold our heads up in the world around us.

Alcoholism is not only rooted in low-self worth but actually makes the situation worse by making us feel increasingly worthless. We end up feeling so bad about who we are, what we are doing and what we have done, that we cannot face life, so we keep drinking. For us alcoholics this only gets worse and never gets better unless we seek and find recovery at depth.

By this, I mean deep change as we allow ourselves to jettison the false beliefs and negative scripts that we have come to believe about ourselves. This is not an overnight job as many of us have been believing self-destructive lies about ourselves from our earliest days. It is difficult to get rid of the old script and start working with the new one.

In the depths of our addiction, we can end up believing that we do not deserve to be here at all and that is a dangerous place to be. Deep recovery involves recovering or even discovering for the first time our self-respect. For the first time, we start to really believe that we are okay and that we are enough rather than less than and not good enough.

As I grow out of my addiction, I am discovering self-respect and a sense of worth as a person that I never knew before. This inner sense of being okay is a powerful force in my ongoing recovery as I challenge and demolish the deeply rooted lies that were spoken endlessly over me as a child. These days when I say I am okay I mean it.

12.10 Deep Recovery

I never thought that recovery from alcoholism was such a deep thing. It's not a superficial treatment as it is more like radical surgery. I found myself examining my motives yesterday as I was in a situation where I was thinking about taking some selfish course of action. I became aware that my motives were suspect and indeed wrong as I felt torn between acting on my impulse or resisting its pull. My dubious motive had revealed the intersection and conflict between doing my will or doing the right thing.

When I got home and thought about it, I realised that before recovery I was oblivious to my motives and would never have really questioned myself in this way. I would have done what I wanted to do without any regard or thought that I might be stepping outside the will of God. I would have unquestioningly gone my way and no doubt got myself and a load of other people into trouble of one sort or another.

Recovery is that deep. It demands rigorous honesty and integrity from me in every area of my life. This was not a drinking issue but my recovery reaches into every area and detail of my thinking and conduct. Unchecked this motive could have led to actions that could have undermined my recovery and the recovery of others.

The discovery of my motives is part of the brave new world of my recovery and it is an exciting one as I learn to live in this world in the way that I was meant to.

12.11 Juvenile Delinquent

Alcoholism meant that my juvenile delinquency continued far longer than it should have done. As long as I was doing the wrong thing with alcohol it opened the door for doing the wrong thing in many other areas of my life. It meant that I could easily make very poor choices and go the wrong way.

When I finally put my drinking in Gods hands, I found that my inner confusion and disorder started to get sorted out. I've heard it said that in recovery we find God doing for us what we could never do for ourselves and this has been true for me. I am now much less likely to make poor choices based on short term selfishness in the way I did when I was drinking.

Things come together for me now in ways that they never did before. Life makes much more sense to me now that I have given up my life as a juvenile delinquent. My alcoholic drinking resulted in a form of arrested development as it held me in a juvenile state. In this condition, I just could not make sense of life in the way that I do now.

The remarkable thing about my recovery is that at last life seems to be working for me. Perhaps this is because I am now working for life rather than against it. Instead of living in the disharmony and disorder of alcoholism, I am enjoying the positive results of seeking to live the right way and doing the right thing in every area of my life.

12.12 Detaching from The Church

As an alcoholic and as the adult child of an alcoholic I had the tendency to become over-attached to certain people. Not only did I become too attached to people but I also became over-attached to the church. In the language of recovery, I became codependent on the church. My life became so tied to the church and its life that I lost myself in it.

Along with drinking my church work came first. I always prioritised it over and above myself and my family. My well being was closely bound up with the well-being of the church. If things were going well in the church, I felt good but if things were going badly, I took it so personally and I would feel deeply unhappy. I had attached my self-worth and indeed my whole life to the well being and prosperity of the church.

It is only in recovery that I have been learning to detach from the church and to realise that I no longer need to attach my life and my well being to its fate. Before recovery, it was a matter of life or death to me but now I have been letting go.

I care deeply about the church and I love it but I have had to detach and let go of the idea that I can control it and make it what I would like it to be. It will be what it will be and there is nothing that I can do about it.

It's not easy to let go but my attempts to control it were just making me ill and for a long time, I used alcohol to relieve the frustration of it all.

12.13 Zombies

I was in town the other day and in front of me were two men who were walking along the street looking like zombies. I realised that they were suffering from the effects of taking a particular street drug that turns them into something like a character from a living dead movie. They were pretty scary and menacing so I avoided them.

That afternoon I had been helping in our local drug and alcohol detox centre and it just so happened that most of the clients I had been with were in a similar state. I had been trying to run a recovery discussion group but it had been difficult because half of them were semi-conscious as they were on high doses of sedatives to prevent withdrawal seizures.

I have seen friends of mine cook their brains on drugs and drink with the result that their previous intelligence had been destroyed and they have been left mentally impaired. We may not get that far but drinking does eventually take its toll on our mental capabilities. Thankfully the human brain is very forgiving and has an enormous capacity for repair and regeneration.

Since stopping drinking alcohol I have noticed that my thinking is much sharper and faster. I have been able to study, research and write with a renewed clarity as a result of having an absolutely clear mind.

I am thankful that I stopped in time so that I have not had to suffer the loss of my mind.

12.14 Social Batteries

In recovery, I have learned to accept myself and not to ignore my own needs as a person. I need lots of time on my own. I need my own space and that is okay.

Knowing, accepting, and living in the light of this means that I don't overextend myself with a social life that I can't manage.

I used to cope with this by using alcohol to get me through but now that I don't drink, I have developed a different approach which involves being realistic about how much socialising I can cope with. My social batteries run out fast and I quickly get exhausted in social situations where I have to be with people for extended periods of time.

I need to pull away to recharge and this is okay. I know myself and I know when I have reached my limits. Knowing this also affects the way that I plan my days and the work that I do. I get my energy from being on my own not from being with other people. So, I have to build lots of time into my schedule for this.

I have noticed that my anxiety levels increase when I see my diary getting too full with social engagements and work events that involve mixing with people. I start to panic because I feel that I will suffocate under the pressure of these social engagements. I find them exhausting and I need to build in lots of time and space between them so that I can recover my breath.

It can be difficult for other people to understand or accept this particularly if they have large social batteries and get their energy from being with people.

12.15 All the Answers

I don't have all the answers to my alcoholism or my alcoholic disposition. I am continuing to gain understanding as life brings challenges and situations to me that force me to search deeper within for the answers.

As a priest people have a tendency to treat me like a slot machine. They feed me their problem or issue and then expect me to come up with the answer immediately. I can't do that for them or even myself. I will never in this lifetime be able to understand or resolve all my own personal issues let alone theirs.

Each of us has our own work and that will always be a work in progress. Life alerts me to my unfinished business as I find myself reacting and responding to my internal as well as my external world.

There is a sense in which my life is a laboratory in which I am carrying out experiments. Some of them go well and others fail. I learn through my failure just as much as through my success.

It is often my failures and problems that hold the key to my growth as I work on them with the help of God and with the counsel of others from within my fellowship. I also exercise patience with myself and no longer demand instant answers and explanations from myself.

12.16 Humility

For me, humility is the recognition that I am no better or no worse than anyone else. It is a recognition and acceptance of my humanity. I am just like everyone else in the human family. We are all in the same boat called life.

Keeping this perspective helps me to walk through life in a way that is of maximum benefit to the people around me. Instead of creating trouble and problems caused by egotistical living, I try to walk humbly with my God. I am not superior or inferior, I am just like every other human being on this planet.

Everything I have is a gift from God so there is little room for boasting about what I have or what I can do. I am a part of rather than apart from the rest of humanity. I believe that I am here to give rather than just to take. I can live unselfishly as day by day I seek to live in the will of God.

And of course, for me as an alcoholic that means not drinking alcohol. From that first step of humble obedience flows everything else that is positive and good in my life.

12.17 Keeping Busy

It is generally recognised that in early recovery it can be a good idea to keep busy so that our minds are distracted from our thoughts about drinking. I was fortunate enough to be able to study for a research degree in my early recovery and it provided a wonderful alternative focus that took my mind right off alcohol. One of my friends started a catering business and another took up wood carving.

In the Alcoholics Anonymous program, we are encouraged to get busy helping other alcoholics as part of our own recovery program and this is all for the good. Sitting around on our own with nothing to do is a bad idea for a newly recovered alcoholic as our minds are prone to take us to some very unhelpful places.

As I have progressed in my recovery, I no longer need to keep busy all the time. What I need to learn now is to be still and to spend time doing nothing in particular. As part of my recovery, I need to learn to switch off and stop my ceaseless activities and busyness. One of the things that helps me is the short silence at the beginning of recovery meetings. It has been a good start as I have often longed for it to go on for longer.

The discipline of stillness and silence reminds me that I am not my mind. My mind is a useful tool but it can be a tyrannical master if I don't learn to keep it in its rightfull place. Silence is one of the ways that I can realise afresh that I am not my mind. As the thoughts race across my consciousness, I am reminded that I don't have to follow them. I can let them pass and be at peace. This is not an instant thing as it can take time for me to relax and take it easy in this way.

Someone once said to me that I should beware of the barrenness of a busy life and now I understand what they mean. Keeping busy or being busy is not an end in itself. I need times of rest and relaxation where my mind can be stilled and I can let go.

12.18 Strange Magic

I have a strong desire to help other alcoholics. It's a strange thing but I am motivated to do anything I can to help those who are still suffering from this disease. I want to help others because I know how much I have been helped by my fellow alcoholics. I also know that in helping others I help myself in the process of staying sober and building a stronger recovery.

There is a strange magic about one alcoholic helping another alcoholic to recover. I am not a health professional but what I have to offer is my own experience, strength and hope to those who are wanting to break free from alcoholism.

It seems that helping other alcoholics is almost always inconvenient but the more I put myself out the more effective my help becomes. I am not an expert but I know that if I place myself at the disposal of my higher power, I will be used to help other alcoholics.

When I help others, I get far more back than I give. It seems that the more I invest in others recovery the greater the return in the depth of my own recovery. It is strange magic because I can't outgive God and the more I give the more I get. If I hold back, it is me who loses out.

Helping others breaks me out of the bondage to self that is such a dangerous aspect of alcoholism.

12.19 More Than My Mind

In recovery, I have become increasingly aware that I am more than my mind. My mind is a useful and good instrument but it is not fully reliable. It can give false readings and take me way off course.

I am more than my best thinking and my way of seeing reality can be very wide of the mark. Ungoverned, my mind can take me in directions that are quite wrong. My mind doesn't like being challenged because it wants to get its own way. It is too easily ruled and dominated by my ego.

I often encounter situations where my mind is wrong and I have to change it. I had to change my mind about alcohol. My ego backed up by my mind said that it was okay for me to drink but this way of thinking was eventually proved to be wrong.

Today as I walk in recovery, I reserve the right to be wrong. When I was drinking, I was not in my right mind but I believed its lies because I wanted to. I deceived my self and the prime suspect in this process was my ego-controlled mind.

I have to constantly keep in mind that I am more than my mind. Left to its own devices it can run riot, so I need to police it and not let it run the show.

12.20 Access All Areas

Just as alcohol affected every area of my life so recovery reaches into all areas and aspects of my living and being. Nothing is off-limits as I continue this journey into life.

Recovery is not a separate compartment but part of every aspect of the way I think and live. Everything in my life comes under its jurisdiction. Any area of my life that I am keeping to myself is a potential danger zone for me. These marshlands of my character are a clue to where I need to do more work.

My areas of personal resistance highlight the things that are in need of attention. They are warning signs that all is not well in this particular area of my life. These areas for attention require me to be honest with myself and not to pretend that all is well when it is not.

Recovery is not about drinking it's about living the best life that I can.

12.21 Free Recovery

The good news is that you don't need to have money to get recovery from alcoholism. Recovery is free and although it can be a good idea to get medically supervised alcohol detoxification the Alcoholics Anonymous recovery program is absolutely free.

There are no fees or subscriptions for this program of recovery. Nobody gets paid for the work and no one is taking money to help you. There are no paid professionals who are making a career out of your problem. There are no forms to fill in or grants to be accessed.

No one asks anything of you and you don't even need to reveal your name. No one tells you what to do and everything you hear is a suggestion with no one keeping score on your progress. You don't have to move out of your accommodation or give up your job if you have one.

You get free tea, coffee and biscuits and if you smoke someone may even give you a cigarette! It's a genius program because you don't need anything to get in except a desire to stop drinking. It doesn't even need to be a consistent desire just a desire and that is all.

Recovery is absolutely free in Alcoholics Anonymous.

12.22 Self-Preservation Society

As I seek to serve and help others I continually hit up against a major obstacle. That obstacle is me and my own self-centred and self-seeking disposition. My internal self-preservation society is very active as it constantly protects my self-interests and wants.

My ego is constantly seeking to take charge so that my future, my finances, my success, my relationships and my needs come first. Left to my own devices my default position is always me.

It is as I reach out to help and serve others that I hit up against this powerful force of resistance within myself. I find myself struggling to help others because I am so wrapped up in myself. I am in bondage to myself.

At the beginning of every day, I now pray that God will deliver me from this bondage to self so that I can break free from its chains and be kind and loving towards all.

I ask God to do what I cannot do for myself which is to change my default setting from me to you and to Him.

12.23 Living in the Solution

I am no longer living in the problem of alcoholism I am living in the solution. I am investing my life in helping myself and others to live in such a way that we work through the problems that arise as we move away from the drinking life.

I meet a lot of people in the detox centre who don't really have an escape plan. Being physically separated from alcohol is one thing but living free is quite another. It requires a program and the willingness to embrace a spiritual way of life that is alien to most alcoholics and addicts.

Many reject this route and some find other ways out of the cycle of addiction but two-thirds of the people I see in detox return to their established patterns of destructive drinking. I am powerless over alcohol and its powers of persuasion are far stronger than mine. All I have is my story of living in the solution and not picking up a drink one day at a time.

I also know that I am not alone and that there is a power that is greater than myself. At the end of the day, it is He and not me who keeps me sober. It is this simple solution that I am seeking to give away to all who really want it.

12.24 My Own Agenda

My will was nailed to drinking. I wanted to drink when, where and how I chose to. My attitude was that it is my life and I have the right to live it just the way I want to. I ran my life on the basis of self-will and even though I had faith it was still deeply rooted in self-serving plans and goals.

It is only as I have been seeking to pursue God's agenda and plan for my life that I have discovered just how deviant I am when it comes to wanting to get my own way and to ignore God.

Behind my plans is a basic fear and insecurity that if I leave it to God, he will not take my life forward in the way that I want it to go. I have a deep-seated sense that God will lead me into difficult and uncomfortable situations that I would rather avoid.

At heart, I don't really believe in God's goodness towards me. I still have my former suspicions that God is actually not on my side and if I go with him then my life will be rough.

Behind this fear and insecurity is the idea of a God who can not be trusted to look after my interests. A God who will let me down and drop me in it so I had better look after myself. It is a manifestation of a lack of basic trust in God.

Because I can't fully trust God not only do I need to be in control of my destiny but I actually find myself thinking that he won't see or won't notice my self-centred schemes and plans that I pursue as I look after myself. I believe that I can just slip my self-serving will in under God's radar even if it involves being disloyal to Him or anyone else.

As I engage in the process of recovery these self-deceptive and self-serving plans and agendas are uncovered and I have the opportunity to take corrective action by not following them and seeking instead to obey God.

12.25 The Impossibility of God

For many of the people that I meet in the detox centre the idea of God is at first glance an impossible one. Their problem with God often arises from the inherited idea of an angry God who is in the business of judgment, punishment and vengeance. This is not a promising place from which to start thinking about God so I try to help my fellow alcoholics to see that this notion of an angry God may not be the most useful one for them to hold onto in recovery.

It turns out that the experience of many addicts and alcoholics is peppered with glimpses of God's goodness, protection and care. Reflection on the circumstances of admission to detox often has an element of miracle about it.

The idea that somebody up there loves me is not so far fetched after all. There just seem to be too many coincidences and lucky breaks for there to be nobody out there, up there or just here.

Even in the depths of alcoholic self-destruction, there are more than a few tales of the intervention of a higher power. Failed suicide attempts and miraculous escapes from the most impossible situations are common amongst those in detox and recovery.

A little thought and some brief discussions soon unearth a wealth of experience of a loving higher power who is on our side and seeking to help us out of the depths of trouble brought on by addiction to alcohol and many other things besides.

It seems that God is not such an impossibility after all.

12.26 I Was Wrong

How powerful these words are for me when I say them and mean them as they reveal true spiritual growth. They are my admission of the defectiveness of my own ego-driven opinions and judgment.

When I say I was wrong and really mean it what I am demonstrating is that I have identified and outed my own self-centred need to be right. I have confronted my human default programming which needs to play God. I have located my prejudice and the conviction that my judgements are right. I am challenging my absolute certainty that the way I see it is the way it is.

These days I reserve the right to be wrong. I am not God and I can't possibly understand everything that goes into making something the way it is. I also can't understand people because we are highly complex and a lot of the time, we can't even understand ourselves.

When I confess that I was wrong I am being honest with myself, with another person and with God.

This is a very healthy way for me to live as I jettison my personal prejudices and judgments that are often the outward manifestation of my underlying resentments and anger.

In recovery, I am seeking to be less opinionated and more open to the idea that my best thinking is fallible and often just plain wrong.

12.27 In My Opinion

Living in my opinion is a very dangerous place for me to be as an alcoholic. When I feel that people have not taken on board my opinion in the form of my advice or proposal then I can easily get the hump. The hump ferments and becomes a powerful brew of bitterness and resentment. All because I had an opinion!

In recovery, I have fewer and fewer opinions as they are too expensive for my emotional and spiritual health. It's alright with me if I don't get my way or don't feel that I have been listened to. People ignore my advice all the time and that's okay.

I am not God and I am far from infallible. The truth is that often I don't know the answer and that's okay. Only God knows the answers to so many of life's questions which is why I keep deferring to him.

These days I pause, pray for wisdom and wait for some sort of answer before offering my opinion.

12.28 Life Happens

When I started out on a six-year-long PhD project my supervisor said something that was really important and that has stuck in my mind ever since. He said that we would have to come to negotiate the fact that life happens and that this would be one of the main challenges for us as we embarked on such an extended period of study.

During those six years, life really did happen for me. I came into recovery from alcoholism, my children left home, my dad became seriously ill and died, I had a stroke and my dog died. I had to keep going with my research even though I felt like I should put it on hold until all these things were dealt with. What I realised was the truth of what my tutor had said which is that life happens.

Even now I can't stop or put the brakes on life because it keeps happening. My recovery has to deal with life on life's terms and sometimes those terms are hard to cope with. Thankfully I now have a lot of support in place when things get tough and I have a relationship with my Higher Power who is looking after me especially when life gets difficult and complicated.

When life happens, I am no longer alone or dependent on a drink and for that I thank God.

12.29 Coming Out Alcoholic

Writing and publishing my confessions means that I will be coming out as an alcoholic. It is not something that I take lightly as the stigma that surrounds the alcoholic label still has some potency. I am so much more than an alcoholic and my own sense of identity is much broader than alcoholism.

However, like a lot of other people who are coming out about their identity in different ways, I am actually proud to be an alcoholic. If I were still drinking, I would not be writing these confessions because I would most likely still be in denial.

I am proud of all the alcoholics who are at this very moment working away at their recovery as they practice the principles and steps of Alcoholics Anonymous. I feel honoured to be part of this most extraordinary fellowship that has provided a way out of addiction for millions of people across the globe.

It is a truly remarkable and miraculous spiritual program and I am proud to be able to shed some more light on it as I reflect on my own experience especially from the perspective of the priesthood.

Confession is a risky business and it never feels comfortable but if it helps others who are struggling with their drinking then I believe that coming out about my own battle with the booze is worthwhile.

12.30 Humbling Myself

I still find it really humbling to have to admit that I am an alcoholic and that I will need to submit to and practice my program of recovery for the rest of my life. No amounts of titles, qualifications or knowledge will let me off the hook. I am just like the street drinkers who I used to encounter every day in the city. I have the same disease and the treatment is the same for me as it is for them.

It's very crushing to my ego and pride to have to acknowledge this but it is the truth. This process of humiliation at the hands of the bottle is not a bad one as it keeps me in check when my ego and pride tempts me to overreach myself. Ego-inflation due to the action of alcohol is no longer a major problem but I need to take care when I find that the ego has landed.

Continued acknowledgement of my alcoholism keeps my feet on the ground and prevents me from excessive pride or an overinflated opinion of myself. Alcoholism is a great leveller. It keeps me rightsized and tends to pierce any bubbles of pride in their earliest stages of development.

12.31 A New Life

My recovery depends on my relationship with God. I no longer depend on other people or my circumstances to keep me sober. As long as I was depending on others my recovery was always on shaky foundations. Good as many people are it had to be me who made the connection with my Higher Power and it has to be me who keeps working on it every day.

This recovery is not just about quitting drinking it's about living my life in a completely different way. It's not the way I used to live. My way wasn't working. My drinking was but a symptom of a deeper disease of the soul.

It is these deep and underlying problems of alcoholism that are now being addressed in recovery. Day by day as I follow my program of recovery and seek to live within rather than outside the will of God, I am finding release and relief from my alcoholic symptoms.

Life gets better now and not worse. I am living a new and different life in recovery. It is a season of new beginnings and real hope that is rooted in reality.

I now look forward to today, tomorrow and next year because I know that if I stay on this pathway things can only get better.

In recovery I have found a new life, I now have hope and a future.

Printed in Great Britain
by Amazon